Welcome to the Wonderful World of GNC

The General Nutrition Corporation, the world's largest firm devoted to nutritious foods and supplements, has satisfied millions of customers for forty-five years. A cornucopia of 2,000 products is sold through mail order and in 800 retail stores throughout the country—and both outlets are steadily expanding. Founder and Chairman David B. Shakarian's inspired idea of farm field to retail store all under one corporate roof carries with it a responsibility for integrity that has never relaxed.

Of the 5,000 employees working toward America's healthkeeping through nutritious foods, none has been more dedicated than Mr. Shakarian, an early convert to the theories of Gayelord Hauser. GNC's products as a result are free of the contaminants now proving to be so hazardous to our health. Attention to quality is its hallmark, its perpetual goal is to provide higher nutritional value at the lowest possible cost.

It is not easy to incorporate such vital foods as brewer's yeast, lecithin or vitamin C into today's depleted diet. But GNC found food specialist Myra Cameron to bring a well-rounded, delightful collection of recipes with explanatory nutritional charts which can bring an end to the mystery of how to get the most out of enjoyable food.

With an inspired blending of cooking expertise, sound nutrition, and the skillful use of the GNC family of vitamins, mineral supplements, natural flours and seasonings, Myra Cameron and your General Nutrition Center present a unique approach to gourmet cuisine—so good it's hard to believe it's good for you!

Books for Better Health at GNC

THE GNC
Gourmet Vitamin Cookbook

**With directions for conventional
and microwave cooking**

MYRA CAMERON
Introduction by BEATRICE TRUM HUNTER

Keats Publishing, Inc.　　New Canaan, Connecticut

THE GNC GOURMET VITAMIN COOKBOOK

Pivot Original Health Book Edition published 1980

Copyright © 1980 by Myra Cameron

All Rights Reserved

No part of this book may be copied or reproduced in any form without the written permission of the publishers.

ISBN: 0-87983-159-6

Library of Congress Catalog Card Number: 80-83226

Printed in the United States of America

Pivot Original Health Books are published by
Keats Publishing, Inc., 36 Grove Street
New Canaan, Connecticut 06840

Contents

Introduction

"HOW IS THIS COOKBOOK different from other cookbooks?" is a justified question posed by potential book buyers, weary of the replicas of standard works, or gimmicky spin-offs. *The GNC Gourmet Vitamin Cookbook* is distinctly different from other cookbooks. Myra Cameron has created recipes using wholesome traditional basic food ingredients, and by adding supplements, has given food dishes extra nutritional boosts. The resulting dishes are gourmet, not hairshirt.

The author dispels the myth that food preparation from scratch needs to be time consuming and laborious. By using modern devices such as an electric food processor, blender, mixer and microwave oven, dishes can be prepared quickly and easily—in the proverbial three shakes of a lamb's tail (which has generously been sprinkled with toasted wheat germ).

Myra Cameron's incorporation of nutritional supplements into food dishes makes good sense. It is a well established fact that foods suffer nutritional losses from garden to gullet, and these losses are beyond our control. They result from certain growing practices, such as picking immature fruits and melons; shipping practices such as cross-country trucking of produce; and storing practices in warehouses and supermarkets. Then, our food may suffer additional decline within our homes, due to improper storage at inappropriate temperatures, and improper handling such as grating, mashing, mauling, overcooking and the cardinal sin of discarding nutrient-rich cooking water. Although each practice may represent only a small nutrient loss, when totalled, they may be significant. We need to be aware of such losses, attempt to minimize them by careful food preparation, and give added boosts to food with beneficial nutrient-rich ingredients whenever we can. Myra Cameron does this by adding such nutritional supports as brewer's yeast powder, bone meal, non-instant powdered milk, whey powder and other beneficial substances.

Another unique feature of this cookbook is an inclusion of comparison charts. For example, the nutrient composition of the author's mayonnaise-like recipe, "Almost Mayonnaise" is contrasted with commercial mayonnaise; "Almost Ice Cream," with commercial ice cream; and a "Super-Nutrition Potato Salad" with a basic potato salad recipe and its commercial counterpart. At times, the "Almost . . ." recipes are useful replacers for commercial products, such as "Almost Maple Syrup" as a satisfactory and less costly substitute for pure maple syrup.

Incorporating nutrition supplements into savory dishes yield certain benefits, in additional to values readily perceived. Supplements are absorbed and utilized best when ingested with food. For this reason, it is usually recommended that supplements in tablet or capsule form be eaten at mealtimes. Certain nutrients can enhance utilization of nutrients, such as better utilization of iron in the presence of ascorbic acid. By incorporating supplements into food dishes, they can be used regularly. This is a special boon to the forgetful. For the member of the family who balks at the idea of pill popping, the incorporation of supplements into food dishes is an immediate, subtle solution, while long-range educational attempts can be made to view supplements as concentrated food. Incorporating food supplements into dishes makes entertaining easier. It eliminates the need to explain the presence of those little tablets next to the dinner plate.

Myra Cameron, who previously authored *Home-style*

Microwave Cooking, provides in *The GNC Gourmet Vitamin Cookbook* specific information for microwave and traditional cookery for recipes that require heat. Experiments have demonstrated that, due to the rapidity of microwave cookery, nutrients are well retained. And the unfounded myth needs to be dispelled that microwave cooking somehow harms food. As a matter of fact, the microwave oven can be used to destroy bacteria on fresh meat and poultry. For example, newly purchased fresh meat, placed in a microwave oven for ten seconds, will keep refrigerated a day or two longer than usual. Microwave ovens are not new. Both food processors and the food service industry have been using them successfully for more than a quarter of a century. What is new is the relatively recent introduction of microwave ovens in American homes. By 1980, more than a quarter of all homes in the United States had microwave ovens.

The GNC Gourmet Vitamin Cookbook combines the best of food ingredients, with an awareness for the need to conserve and increase nutrient values, and offers the means for quick, easy food preparation. These three elements combine to make this cookbook unique and helpful.

Beatrice Trum Hunter

A Note from
Myra Cameron

WITHOUT attempting to play favorites among the countless diet and nutritional philosophies currently in vogue, this book offers an immediate and positive solution for bringing our overly refined, processed and preserved diets up to ideal nutritional standards.

The wealth of natural supplements offered by GNC is combined in easily prepared dishes with the marvelous variety of foods now available the year around to let us enjoy the best of both worlds: *old-fashioned* nutrition and *modern* technology.

Food preparation can be a wonderfully satisfying, creative hobby; but few of us have time to savour the enjoyment; busy schedules seldom include time for shelling peas on the front porch or allowing bread to rise for two hours after a ten-minute hand kneading. By using electric blenders or processors, instant liquid tenderizer, microwave ovens or pressure cookers for quick cooking, and a touch of vitamin C powder, kelp or sea salt for seasoning, we can serve nutrition-packed meals with less time and effort than preparing packaged mixes.

The recipes are tailored to fit today's small families, with four servings of most foods, six for those especially suitable for guests or for planned-over leftovers, and an occasional quantity-recipe for large groups or for stocking the freezer. Preparation methods also are adjusted for current lifestyles and the assumption that all family members are away from home for eight or nine hours each day. Even the long-soaking and slow-cooking timings are compatible with this schedule, with none of the traditional "over-night" instructions as so few of us are available for the "next morning" follow-up. Note that ingredients shown in caps may be obtained through GNC.

GNC offers whole-grain flours (with all 23 of the nutrients instead of the six replaced in "enriched" commercial flour*) or you can use a small, electric seed grinder for freshly-ground wheat or rye flour to make yeast bread so quickly and easily it seems almost sinful. Nutritional yeast, wheat germ, lecithin, and cold-pressed oils provide even more of the B-complex and vitamin E than our grandmothers' breads, while a bit of powdered dolomite and bone meal furnish the calcium, magnesium and phosphorus of a quart of milk per loaf; and skim milk powder, gluten and soy flours add protein without excess calories.

You will notice that many of the recipes are followed by a variation for SUPER-NUTRITION for those who have had additional vitamins and minerals recommended by their physicians. Any or all of the supplements may be used as shown without altering the flavor of the recipe. There are also recipes for "emergency rations"—snack-type foods that can be kept in the refrigerator and/or freezer.

In addition to better health from better nutrition, there is a pleasant bonus to cooking-with-vitamins—it saves money! GNC supplements cost far less than either the natural foods or the capsules required to provide the equivalent in essential nutrients, and complete proteins are less expensive when grains and legumes are included as part of the team.

Good nutrition cannot be built on pills alone; the human body requires the components of "real food" in order to perform its chemical miracles. But even a diet of real foods (foods in their natural state, untampered with by man) cannot assure us of even the Recommended Daily

---

Mega Nutrients for Your Nerves by Dr. Newbold, Berkley Publishing Corp. N.Y. 1978.

Allowance (RDA) of the needed nutrients—let alone provide the extras to take care of added stress, exertion, illness, harmful chemicals in the air and water, or existing nutritional deficiencies. All produce suffers vitamin and mineral losses before it reaches our kitchens. Vitamin C disappears from cabbage in three days after picking, and the average time from picking to produce counter is six days.* Potatoes lose one-fourth of their vitamin C when stored for one month, three-fourths if stored for nine months. Regardless of the care with which food is prepared, further losses occur—a potato baked in its skin loses 21 percent of its remaining vitamins, and 49 percent when peeled and cooked in water. Even greater losses occur once the food is eaten—only 1 percent of the carotene in a raw carrot is absorbed as vitamin A in the body, up to 35 percent when cooked and pureed with the cooking liquid.

The Nutritional Analysis Tables are based on the nutritive value of foods as given in the *USDA Handbook #8* with supplements, and *Nutrition Almanac* by Nutrition Search Inc. These figures represent the amount of nutrients in the foods when prepared—not the amount assimilated—so the need for supplements is obvious. A list of supplements and ingredients precedes the analysis tables; GNC order numbers are given.

Diet Revolution by Jill Wordsworth, St. Martin's Press, N.Y. 1977.

MICROWAVE COOKING DIRECTIONS are for a 650-watt, counter-top microwave oven without a rotating turn-table, and call for only the full power (High) or half power (Defrost) settings. Cooking times would need to be increased by approximately one third for 400 to 500-watt ovens and can vary with fluctuations of house current as well as the type of container used and the temperature of ingredients. (The cardinal rule for all microwave cooking is to under-cook and test.) If your oven has a carousel, omit the instructions for turning the dishes while cooking and add a few seconds to the cooking time to compensate for the continued cooking that would have taken place during manual turning.

CHAPTER 1
Soups

HOMEMADE BROTHS and stocks are a key factor in vitamin-enriched, gourmet-style cooking, and generations of intuitive cooks have unknowingly aided their families' nutrition by keeping a soup pot simmering on the back of the stove.

Meat and poultry bones and trimmings contain a wealth of minerals and when vegetables are chopped, simmered and allowed to stand for a few minutes, as much as 90 percent of their vitamin and mineral content passes into the cooking liquid. Of all the known vitamins, only vitamin C and folic acid are harmed by boiling temperature (212 degrees F.), vitamin B_1 is destroyed only when held at a temperature well above boiling, and all of the minerals safely dissolve in water.*

There are countless recipes for making broths from freshly purchased supplies, but with our modern freezers we can accomplish the same delicious results at practically no cost by utilizing meat and vegetable trimmings. By maintaining three plastic bags in an easily accessible freezer you can stockpile ingredients for these money-saving broths and at the same time up-grade your meats and glamorize your vegetables. Gourmet foods aren't necessarily odd or expensive, but they must be delicious and attractive.

When you are "saving for the soup pot" you can trim with a clear conscience, knowing that the food value, vitamins and minerals will all be put to good use. Celery strings and tops, woody mushroom stems, wilted lettuce

---

Let's Cook It Right by Adelle Davis, Harcourt, Brace, Jovanovich, N.Y. 1970.

3

leaves or carrot peelings; chicken skin, necks, backs and wings; meat bones, gristle and membrane all can accumulate in their separate bags while you serve delectable, presentation-perfect meals. Food is sterilized at 140 degrees F., so even the most particular need have no compunction about salvaging steak or chicken bones from dinner plates. And, if there is a half-glass of tomato juice or some liquid remaining with cooked vegetables, it can be frozen in a small container and popped into the vegetable-broth bag.

The time-proven method of slowly simmering a large pot of beef or chicken stock is still practical during cold weather, and imparts a heart-warming aroma to the kitchen. Vegetable broth should be cooked more quickly to retain vitamins and avoid the strong or bitter flavor-change which occurs in overcooked vegetables containing sulfur. A few minutes of boiling in a covered saucepan, or even fewer in a pressure cooker or microwave oven, will suffice. When extra kitchen heat is not appreciated, a slow-cooker, pressure cooker or microwave oven can be used for cooking the meat or poultry broths.

In addition to the time and bother saved by modern appliances, there are a few trouble-saving tricks to take the rest of the work out of broth making:

1. Increase the ratio of solid ingredients to liquid to make a large quantity of broth in a small cooking container. This not only shortens the cooking time, but produces double-strength broths which require little freezer space and are the equivalent of canned, condensed broths or consommés for cooking purposes, but much more potent nutritionally.
2. Chill cooked, strained meat or poultry broths to avoid any skimming of foam or fat. The foam that rises to the surface during cooking contains valuable nutrients that will settle to the bottom of the cold liquid. Fats will rise to the top and form a firm layer which can be lifted

off to leave a clear, rich broth, usually semi-solid when chilled because of the unrefined gelatin from the bones. The cloudy layer in the bottom can be utilized in meat loaves or casseroles so no food value is wasted.

3. Freeze the clear broth in small containers for quick defrosting and convenience for countless uses beyond the making of soup.

VEGETABLE BROTH

The quickest and easiest of all, vegetable broth requires no chilling before use and adds both flavor and nutrients to soups, sauces and vegetable-juice beverages. It may even be used as the liquid for cooking other vegetables, potatoes, rice or macaroni— and it is free for the making!

Potato peelings would cloud the broth so they should be reserved for making potato chips according to the recipe on page 61. Beets would over-color it and too large a proportion of turnips or cabbage would overpower it—but all other vegetables may be included. Wash vegetables and cut out any blemished portions before preparing them for salads or cooking, then hoard everything from the ends of asparagus stalks to zucchini seeds. Parsley stems, carrot tops and radish bottoms add interest. If you have a juice extractor, you can extract the final nutrients from the pulp it ejects when making vegetable liquids by adding it to the accumulation.

If your storage bag is filled before any onions, tomatoes or carrots are included, add one-half cup of each chopped vegetable when making the broth to assure flavor and nutritional balance.

4 to 6 cups chopped vegetables and trimmings	½ teaspoon SEA SALT
½ teaspoon KELP	¼ teaspoon FRUCTOSE GRANULES

Partially defrost the frozen vegetables, then chop by hand or in a food processor. Place in a saucepan and cover with hot tap water. Add kelp, salt and fructose. Cover and bring to boiling over high heat. Stir, reduce heat and boil slowly for 15 minutes. Let stand for 30 minutes.

WITH MICROWAVE OVEN: Place the partially defrosted, chopped vegetables in a 2-quart casserole. Add kelp, salt, fructose, and enough hot tap water to cover the vegetables. Microwave, covered, for 15 minutes on full power—stirring each 5 minutes. Let stand 30 minutes.

WITH PRESSURE COOKER: Place the partially defrosted and chopped vegetables in the pressure cooker. Add kelp, salt and fructose. Pour in hot tap water to cover the vegetables. Close the cover and put the pressure control in place. When full pressure is reached, cook for 7 minutes. Let the pressure go down of its own accord and leave the vegetables in the cooker for about 20 minutes.

Strain into a mixing bowl and press to remove the liquid without forcing the pulp through the sieve. Store in the refrigerator or freeze in small containers.

BEEF BROTH

Soup bones once were given away at meat counters but now are so expensive it pays to grow your own. Not by going into the cattle-raising business, but by freezing the bones and trimmings from round steaks or flat roasts before cooking or packaging them for the freezer, and by retrieving the bones from cooked meats. (The simmering broth sterilizes!) When meat has been frozen "bone-in" it is wise to cook the bones before re-freezing them. Do this by baking in a hot oven or browning in a skillet or microwave browning dish to avoid any possibility of bacterial contamination and to add an appetizing color to the broth.

Pork or veal bones may be included with either beef or chicken bones, and any less expensive (the word used to be "cheap") cut of meat may be added to enrich the broth and provide succulently tender cooked beef with the same expenditure of energy. Drippings from meat loaves and oven roasts may be included if they are first chilled so the layer of fat can be removed, then frozen and added to the growing bag of bones.

A little acid, in the form of apple cider vinegar, lemon juice or wine, will hasten the breakdown of connective tissue and dissolve the calcium from the bones. A few vegetables should be added for flavor and vitamins but no specific formula need be followed. The following recipe gives proportionate amounts.

Beef plus defrosted bones and trimmings (no solid fat) to fill a 3- or 4-quart cooking container ⅔ full

1 medium carrot, chopped

½ medium onion, studded with 2 whole cloves

2 leafy celery tops

2 slices turnip or 2 sliced radishes (or the equivalent in trimmings)

2 tablespoons snipped parsley (or the equivalent in parsley stems)

1 chopped tomato or ½ cup tomato juice

2 tablespoons APPLE CIDER VINEGAR

2 teaspoons SEA SALT

1 teaspoon KELP SEASONING

¼ teaspoon whole peppercorns

Place bones, meat, vegetables and seasonings in cooking container. Add hot tap water to cover. Cover the container and bring to boiling on high heat. Reduce heat to low and simmer for 8 to 12 hours in a large kettle on the stove or in a slow-cooker.

WITH MICROWAVE OVEN: Use a 3- or 4-quart casserole and fill 2/3 full with bones, meat, vegetables and seasonings. Add hot tap water to cover. Microwave on full power for 10 minutes, covered, or until mixture is boiling. Set control on Defrost (half power) and microwave for 90 minutes, turning dish each 30 minutes.

WITH 4- TO 6-QUART PRESSURE COOKER: Place bones, meat, vegetables, seasonings and water in the pressure cooker. Close the cover and set for the lowest pressure. Cook for 1½ hours after the control jiggles. Allow pressure to drop of its own accord.

WITH 2½- TO 3-QUART ELECTRIC PRESSURE COOKER: Fill according to the manufacturer's instructions, reduce seasonings accordingly and cook for 45 minutes under full pressure.

Strain the broth into a bowl and cool immediately by placing the bowl in a larger pan partially filled with cold water and ice cubes. Shred off and reserve any usable meat. Discard the vegetables as even vitamins A, E and K will have leached out into the cooking liquid from the chopped vegetables. Refrigerate the broth 2 to 24 hours so the fat will solidify and can be lifted off and discarded.

To test the broth for strength and flavor, combine 1 teaspoon with 1 teaspoon hot water and taste. If the broth seems weak you can transfer the clear, jellied broth to a saucepan, add salt if needed, and boil rapidly for a few minutes to further condense it. Reserve the cloudy layer at the bottom of the jellied broth for use in meat loaves or casserole dishes. Refrigerate the clear broth for up to three days or freeze it in small containers for longer storage.

Yield: Approximately 5 cups double-strength broth (equal to four 10-ounce cans of condensed beef bouillon)

CHICKEN BROTH

The plastic bag of chicken backs, necks, accumulated skin and bones, wings and giblets (unless enjoyed when cooked separately) plus a few drumstick-thighs for additional shredded chicken, can be transformed into delicious broth by adjusting the seasonings and using the same method as for beef broth.

Chicken plus defrosted bones and skin to fill a 3- or 4-quart cooking container ⅔ full
1 medium carrot, chopped
½ medium onion, chopped
4 leafy celery tops
2 tablespoons snipped parsley (or the equivalent in parsley stems)

2 tablespoons APPLE CIDER VINEGAR
2 teaspoons SEA SALT
1 teaspoon GRANULATED KELP
¼ teaspoon ground white pepper
¼ teaspoon poultry seasoning

Place all ingredients in cooking container, add hot tap water to cover and cook as for Beef Broth.

For regular-strength chicken broth, see the recipe for Delicatessen Chicken on page 100.

MIXED BROTH

Called "brodo" in Italy, mixed broth may be used in place of either beef or chicken broth in soups and cooking. When it's time to clear the freezer or when there isn't enough beef or chicken to warrant cooking them separately, try this easy combination.

Reserved beef, chicken, pork and veal bones and trimmings (no solid fat) to fill a 3- or 4-quart cooking container ⅔ full

2 tablespoons APPLE CIDER VINEGAR
2 teaspoons SEA SALT
1 teaspoon KELP SEASONING Vegetable Broth*

Place all ingredients except vegetable broth in cooking container. Heat broth and add to cover. Cook as for Beef or Chicken Broth.

_____

*If no vegetable broth is on hand, make it from the bag of vegetable trimmings and let it stand while defrosting the meat and poultry. Strain the hot broth into the cooking container over the meat and poultry, vinegar, salt and kelp and proceed as directed. (Or stir Vegetable Salad Powder into hot water to taste.)

COCK-A-LEEKIE (Scottish Chicken Soup)

Chicken breast cooks so quickly that the microwave method of instant preparation can be adapted to stove-top cooking for equally succulent bites of chicken in a soup that is spectacularly high in protein and potassium, plus vitamins A and C.

½ large chicken breast (at least ½ pound before boning and skinning)
1 tablespoon dry white wine or apple juice
1 teaspoon COLD PRESSED ALL BLEND OIL
⅛ teaspoon C-TRATE

3 cups chicken broth (homemade or canned) divided
1 medium carrot
3 tablespoons STEEL CUT OAT-MEAL
2 cups leeks in ¼-inch slices
1 cup peeled, diced potato
¼ teaspoon ground white pepper
¼ teaspoon SEA SALT

Bone and skin chicken breast. Cut into ¾-inch pieces and marinate in the wine, oil and C-Trate. Bring 2 cups of the broth to boiling in a covered saucepan. Pour remaining broth into the container of an electric blender. Peel or scrape carrot and cut in chunks. Add to broth in blender and whirl until quite fine. Empty into the boiling broth and stir in with the oatmeal. (Or grate carrot by hand and stir into the boiling broth with the oatmeal and remaining broth.) Cover and simmer for 15 minutes. Stir in leeks, potato and pepper. Replace cover and simmer until vegetables are tender—about 20 minutes. Stir in chicken, marinade and salt. Cover and simmer 5 minutes, or until chicken is firm and white.

TO MICROWAVE: Bone and skin chicken. Cut into ¾-inch pieces and marinate in the wine, oil and C-Trate. Peel or scrape carrot and cut in chunks. Whirl in an electric blender with 1 cup of broth until quite fine. (Or grate by hand.) Place in a 2-quart casserole and rinse blender (if used) with 1 cup of broth. Stir into the casserole with the oatmeal. Cover and microwave on full power for 10 minutes. (If the broth was chilled, microwave for an additional 2 minutes.) Stir in leeks, potato, pepper and remaining cup of broth. Cover and microwave for 15 minutes on full power. Stir in chicken, marinade and salt. Cover and microwave for 3 minutes. Let stand 2 minutes before serving.

Yield: 4 one-cup servings

CREAM OF LETTUCE & TOMATO SOUP

Garden-fresh flavor in a light cream soup to add a touch of warmth to an otherwise cold summer meal, or to serve whenever leaf lettuce is abundant. Using skim milk powder in place of a flour or starch thickening makes this a high protein soup (over 9 grams per bowl) and adds calcium to its amazing amounts of other minerals and vitamins. Since most of the vitamin C will have been destroyed by the heat of cooking, you may want to stir in a bit of vitamin C powder just before serving.

3 cups shredded or chopped leaf lettuce
1 tablespoon COLD PRESSED ALL BLEND OIL
⅓ cup chopped green onions with crisp tops
1 cup chopped raw tomatoes
2 tablespoons snipped parsley
1 teaspoon SPIKE
3 cups chicken broth (homemade or canned) divided
½ cup non-instant SKIM MILK POWDER

Wash lettuce, dry in a salad spinner or blot with paper towels. Shred in a food processor or chop by hand and combine with the oil and onions in a 2-quart saucepan. Cook and stir for 5 minutes, or until vegetables are limp.

Stir in tomatoes, parsley and Spike, then add half the broth. Cover and bring to a full boil over medium heat. Let stand for 3 minutes.

Measure ½ cup broth in the container of an electric blender, add skim milk powder and blend until smooth. Pour in hot soup and blend on high speed. Return to saucepan. Rinse blender with remaining cup of broth and stir into soup. Heat just to serving temperature, do not boil after adding to milk.

TO MICROWAVE: Wash and dry lettuce. Shred or chop and combine with the oil and onions in a 1½-quart casserole. Cover and microwave on full power for 4 minutes, stirring once. Stir in tomatoes, parsley, Spike and half the broth. Cover and microwave on full power until boiling—about 5 minutes. Let stand for 3 minutes.

Blend skim milk powder with ½ cup broth in an electric blender. Pour in the hot soup and blend on high speed. Return to the casserole. Rinse blender with remaining cup of broth and stir into the soup. Microwave, uncovered, just to serving temperature—3 to 5 minutes depending on the temperature of the broth. Do not boil after adding the milk.

NOTE: To avoid using an electric blender, combine skim milk powder with ½ cup broth in a mixing bowl and blend with an egg beater. Puree the cooked lettuce, onions and broth by pressing through a sieve or using a food mill.

Yield: 4 one-cup servings

HOTCH-POTCH (Scottish Oatmeal Soup)

This vegetarian adaptation is even thriftier than the original Scottish version which called for lamb neck bones. Oatmeal and dried peas fill the amino acid gaps for each other, increasing their protein value; and replacing the vitamin C lost through cooking makes this delicious soup even more of a nutritional bargain.

1 tablespoon safflower margarine	1 large stalk celery with leaves
1 medium onion, chopped	1 small wedge cabbage
2½ tablespoons (1 ounce) STEEL CUT OATMEAL	1½ teaspoons VEGETABLE SALAD POWDER
3½ cups hot tap water	1 teaspoon SEA SALT
2 tablespoons (1 ounce) dried split peas	1 tablespoon snipped parsley
1 large carrot	¼ teaspoon C-TRATE
½ medium turnip	⅛ teaspoon freshly ground black pepper

Heat margarine in 3-quart saucepan over medium heat. Chop and add onions. Cook and stir for 5 minutes—until limp but not browned. Stir in oatmeal and cook for 1 minute. Add hot water and split peas. Bring to boiling, cover and simmer for 30 minutes. Stir occasionally during the last half of the cooking time. Chop or shred carrot, turnip, celery and cabbage, by hand or with food processor. Stir into the soup with Vegetable Salad Powder and salt. Return to boiling, cover and simmer until all are tender—about 30 minutes. Stir in parsley, C-Trate and black pepper.

WITH MICROWAVE OVEN: Cut margarine in quarters and combine with onion in 2-quart casserole. Microwave on full power, uncovered, for 2 minutes.

Stir in oatmeal, 1½ cups of hot water and the split peas. Cover and microwave 15 minutes on full power, stirring after 10 minutes. Chop or shred carrot, turnip, celery and cabbage, by hand or with a food processor. Stir into the soup with Vegetable Salad Powder, salt and remaining 2 cups hot water. Cover and microwave 15 minutes on full power, stirring after 10 minutes. Stir in parsley, C-Trate and pepper.

WITH PRESSURE COOKER: Heat margarine in 3- or 4-quart open pressure cooker and sauté onion until limp but not browned. Stir in oatmeal and cook for 1 minute. Add hot water and split peas. Close cover and set pressure control in place. When pressure is reached, cook for 10 minutes. Cool cooker at once under running water. Add chopped carrots, turnip, celery and cabbage. Stir in Vegetable Salad Powder and salt. Close cover of cooker and put pressure control in place. When pressure is reached and control jiggles, cook for 10 mintues. Cool at once under running water. Stir in parsley, C-Trate and black pepper.

Yield: 4 servings

WITH SLOW-COOKER: Double the ingredients, let them simmer all day, and eight bowls of soup will be waiting for you at dinner time!

In a small skillet, sauté the onions with the margarine. Stir in the oats and transfer to a 3- or 4-quart slow-cooker. Stir in 7 cups of hot water plus the doubled amounts of all other ingredients except for the parsley, C-Trate and black pepper. Cover and cook on Low for 10-12 hours. Stir in parsley, C-Trate and pepper just before serving.

Any soup not needed immediately may be frozen in 1-cup containers.

Yield: 8 cups soup

LENTIL-BARLEY SOUP

A big, bubbling pot of soup is so nice to come home to—and slow-cookers are even better than the old iron kettles on the farmhouse stoves because they don't destroy the vitamin C and no one has to tend the fire all day! The intriguing blend of flavors in this substantial soup pleases guests as well as family members and the additional protein in the super-nutrition variation qualifies it as the main attraction. Serve with a salad and freshly warmed, homemade bread, then follow with dessert for a memorable meal. The amounts of usable nutrients are also remarkable: lentils and barley complement each other to form complete protein; chopping and simmering the vegetables reduces their vitamin A, and other water-soluble vitamins and minerals, to their most assimilable form; the "balancing acts" of potassium-sodium and magnesium-calcium-phosphorus are in order—and there is even a respectable amount of fiber!

1 cup dry LENTILS	1 large stalk celery with leaves
¼ cup BARLEY	2 cloves garlic
5 cups water	2 cups canned tomatoes (1 16-ounce can)
1 teaspoon INSTANT LIQUID TENDERIZER	1 teaspoon COLD PRESSED SESAME OIL
1 medium onion	
1 tablespoon safflower margarine	2 tablespoons APPLE CIDER VINEGAR
1½ teaspoons SEA SALT	1 tablespoon BLACKSTRAP MOLASSES
1 teaspoon dry mustard	Black pepper
½ teaspoon crushed red pepper	
1 large carrot	

Rinse lentils and place in a 3- or 4-quart saucepan with the barley. Stir in water and tenderizer. Let stand 20 minutes.

While lentils are standing, chop onion by hand or in a food processor and sauté with the margarine until limp but not browned. Stir in salt, mustard and red pepper. Chop carrot, celery and garlic, stir in and cook for 1 minute. Cut tomatoes in bite-sized bits, or process briefly, and stir into the onion-vegetable mixture.

Stir the vegetables into the lentils and barley, add oil,

cover and bring to boiling. Reduce heat and simmer for 45 minutes. Stir in vinegar and molasses. Cover and simmer until all are tender. Additional water and/or salt may be added with the black pepper before serving, if desired.

WITH SLOW-COOKER: Rinse lentils and place in saucepan with barley. Stir in water and tenderizer. Let stand 20 minutes.

While lentils are standing, chop onion by hand or in a food processor and sauté with the margarine until limp but not browned. Stir in salt, mustard and red pepper. Chop carrot, celery and garlic and stir in. Cut tomatoes in bite-sized bits, or process briefly, and stir into the onion-vegetable mixture. Cover and bring to boiling.

Bring lentils to a full boil over medium heat and pour into slow-cooker. Add boiling vegetable mixture. Stir in vinegar, molasses and oil. Cover and cook on Low for 10-12 hours. Stir in additional water and/or salt if desired, and add a sprinkling of freshly ground black pepper just before serving.

SUPER-NUTRITION VARIATION:

- Substitute 5 cups of beef broth for the water and use only 1 teaspoon salt
- Add to the sauteed onions: 2 tablespoons SOY FLOUR
  1 teaspoon BONE MEAL POWDER
  1 teaspoon DOLOMITE POWDER
  1 teaspoon KELP SEASONING
- Just before serving, stir in: 2 tablespoons snipped parsley
  ¼ teaspoon C-Trate

Yield: 8 servings

WITH MICROWAVE OVEN: For the fast microwave version, use half the amount of each ingredient. You'll also need to substitute garlic powder for the garlic cloves and vary the preparation order just a bit.

Combine 2 cups of water with ½ cup rinsed lentils and ½ teaspoon tenderizer in a bowl and let stand 20 minutes.

Chop one-half onion and microwave with 1½ teaspoons margarine in a 2-quart casserole for 1 minute on full power. Stir in 2 tablespoons barley and microwave for 1 more minute. Stir in ¾ teaspoon salt, ½ teaspoon mustard and ¼ teaspoon crushed red pepper. Chop 1 small carrot, 1 small stalk of celery and 1 cup of canned tomatoes. Stir in with ⅛ teaspoon garlic powder. Cover and microwave on full power for 5 minutes.

Stir in lentils, soaking liquid, 1 tablespoon vinegar, 1½ teaspoons molasses and ½ teaspoon sesame oil. Cover and microwave 20 minutes on full power, stirring after 10 minutes. Stir in 1 cup water, cover and microwave for 15 minutes on full power—stirring halfway through the cooking time. (If lentils and barley are still too chewy, microwave an additional 5 minutes.) Stir in additional water, if needed to make 4 cups of soup, and add salt if desired. Sprinkle with freshly ground black pepper and serve to four.

For the SUPER-NUTRITION VARIATION, use half the amounts of soy flour and supplements; add as directed for conventional or slow-cooker soup.

QUICK CHILI WITH BEANS

A quickly prepared, gourmet-style chili; thick, dark and rich (thanks to the carob, blackstrap and lecithin) with authentic south-of-the-border flavor. If it is not prefaced by a bowl of fresh vegetable nibbles with an enriched dairy dip, dolomite and vita-

min C powder could be added to the chili with the beans. (The raw vegetables will qualify as gourmet fare if you refer to them as "crudités"!)

½ pound lean ground beef
½ large onion, chopped (¾ cup)
1 tablespoon SOY FLOUR
1 teaspoon CAROB POWDER
1 teaspoon chili powder*
¾ teaspoon SEA SALT
½ teaspoon KELP SEASONING
⅛ teaspoon *each* garlic powder and ground cumin
1¼ cups canned tomatoes with liquid

1 tablespoon chopped, canned green chiles*
½ cup beef broth (homemade or canned)
1 teaspoon BLACKSTRAP MOLASSES
1 teaspoon LIQUID LECITHIN
2 cups cooked pinto beans with liquid (cooking directions are on page 124)

Sauté beef and onion in a 2-quart saucepan, stirring frequently, until onion is limp but not browned. Blot any fat with a paper towel. Stir in flour, carob, chili powder, salt, kelp, garlic and cumin. Cut up tomatoes and chiles by hand or place in an electric blender or processor and whir for a few seconds. Stir into the meat mixture with the broth. Cover and bring to a boil; lower heat and simmer, stirring occasionally, for 20 minutes. Stir in molasses, lecithin and beans. Heat to serving temperature.

TO MICROWAVE: Combine beef and onion in a 2-quart casserole. Cover with a paper towel and microwave 4 minutes on full power. Blot liquid with the paper towel. Stir in flour, carob, chili powder, salt, kelp, garlic and cumin. Chop tomatoes and chiles (or whirl in an electric blender or processor) and stir into the meat mixture. Cover and microwave on full power for 8 minutes, stirring after 5 minutes. Stir in broth, molasses, lecithin and beans. Cover and microwave on full power for 3 minutes, or until at serving temperature.

Yield: Approximately 5 cups = 4 servings

---

*Additional chili powder and/or green chiles may be added for the aficionados of fiery chili.

17

ROOT CELLAR SOUP

Long before modern processing and refrigerated storage, cool, damp root cellars (usually a sort of cave hollowed out of the earth and fronted with a wooden door) held the winter's supply of root vegetables for each family. Combining some of these vegetables with dried beans and a little meat could, and can, produce delicious, high-protein, high-vitamin fare such as this thick, old-fashioned soup-stew intended for serving over or with bread instead of crackers. Add more beef broth if you prefer a thinner soup.

⅔ cup dry white beans (Great Northern or Navy)

¾ teaspoon INSTANT LIQUID TENDERIZER

3 cups water

¾ pound lean, boneless round steak, cut in half-inch cubes

1 tablespoon COLD PRESSED ALL BLEND OIL

1 medium onion, chopped (1 cup)

¼ cup BARLEY

2 medium rutabagas (½ pound), finely chopped

1 medium carrot, scraped or peeled and finely chopped

¾ cup finely chopped solid cabbage, firmly packed (3½ ounces)

3 cups beef broth (homemade or canned)

1 tablespoon dried parsley

1 teaspoon TAMARI SOY SAUCE

1 teaspoon SEA SALT

1 teaspoon KELP SEASONING

1/16 teaspoon ground red pepper (cayenne)

Wash beans and combine in a kettle with the tenderizer and water. Let stand 5 minutes and bring to a full boil for 2 minutes. Cover and let stand for 1 hour.

Sauté beef cubes in the oil and transfer to the kettle of beans. Add onion to drippings; cook and stir until limp, then stir in barley and cook for 1 minute. Add to the beans. Chop rutabagas, carrot, and core plus some surrounding solid cabbage by hand, in a food processor, or with 1 cup of the broth in an electric blender. Add to beans with broth, parsley, soy sauce, salt, kelp and red pepper. Cover and bring to boiling. Reduce heat and simmer until beans are tender, about 2 hours.

WITH SLOW-COOKER: Prepare soup as directed transferring precooked, soaked beans and sautéed beef, onions and barley to the slow-cooker instead of a kettle. Stir in remaining ingredients, cover and cook on Low for 8 to 12 hours—until beans and barley are tender.

Yield: 8 cups soup = 8 servings

WITH MICROWAVE OVEN: For meaningful time saving, quantities need to be reduced and the preparation order altered. Briefly microwaving the beef cubes results in tender bits of "steak" instead of "stewed" beef.

½ cup dry white beans (Great Northern or Navy)

1 teaspoon INSTANT LIQUID TENDERIZER, divided

2 cups plus 1 tablespoon water, divided

6 ounces lean, boneless round steak in half-inch cubes

1 teaspoon TAMARI SOY SAUCE

½ medium onion (½ cup chopped)

1 teaspoon COLD PRESSED ALL BLEND OIL

2 tablespoons BARLEY

1 medium rutabaga (¼ pound) peeled and finely chopped

1 small carrot, scraped or peeled and finely chopped

⅓ cup finely minced cabbage, firmly packed

2 cups beef broth (home-made or canned) divided

1½ teaspoons dried parsley

½ teaspoon SEA SALT

½ teaspoon KELP SEASONING

pinch ground red pepper (cayenne)

Wash beans and combine with ½ teaspoon tenderizer and 2 cups of water in a 1½-quart cooking dish. Let stand 5 minutes. Cover and microwave on full power until the beans have boiled for 1 minute—a total cooking time of about 6 minutes. Let stand for 1 hour.

In a small dish, combine steak cubes with the tablespoon of water and the soy sauce. Cover and let stand.

Place onion and oil in a 2-quart casserole and microwave, uncovered, for 2 minutes on full power.

19

Stir in barley and microwave for 1 minute. Add soaked beans with their liquid and 1 cup of broth. Cover and microwave on full power for 10 minutes. Stir, set control on Defrost (half power) and microwave for 15 minutes. Chop rutabaga, carrot and cabbage by hand, in a food processor, or with 1 cup of the broth in an electric blender. Stir into the bean mixture with remaining broth, parsley, salt, kelp and red pepper. Cover and microwave on full power for 25 minutes, stirring after 15 minutes. Let stand 5 minutes. (If beans and barley are not tender, microwave for an additional few minutes.)

Spread meat and marinade on a plate, cover with a piece of waxed paper and microwave on full power for 2 minutes. Stir meat and liquid into the soup. Microwave for 2 or 3 minutes if the soup has cooled, but do not boil after adding the meat.

Yield: Approximately 5 cups = 4 servings

SUPER-NUTRITION VARIATION: This soup is fairly bubbling with nourishment, including 16 grams of complete protein per cup. For a meal-in-a-bowl, stir in ¼ teaspoon C-Trate and the contents of a 10,000 IU Super Dry A & D capsule just before serving. (For the microwaved version, use a 5,000 IU capsule and ⅛ teaspoon vitamin C powder.)

SALMON SOUP

More bisque than chowder, this creamy soup with its high protein, calcium and potassium content is ideal for soup-and-salad luncheons or suppers. Little preparation time is required, but to avoid last minute kitchen clutter when serving guests, cook the vegetables, puree them with the skim milk powder and water, and refrigerate. When ready to serve, add the salmon and heat—right in the soup tureen if using microwaves.

1 tablespoon safflower margarine	1 8-ounce can pink salmon, with
1/2 medium onion (1/2 cup chopped)	liquid
1 rib celery, chopped	1/2 teaspoon SEA SALT
1 large potato (1/2 pound) peeled	1/4 teaspoon paprika
1¾ cups water, divided	1/8 teaspoon ground white pepper
⅔ cup non-instant SKIM MILK POWDER	

Sauté onion and celery with margarine in a 2-quart saucepan until the onion is limp. Chop potatoes and add with ¾ cup of the water. Cover and cook over low heat until potatoes are tender—about 15 minutes—stirring occasionally.

Pour the remaining cup of water into the container of an electric blender, add skim milk powder and blend on high speed for 10 seconds. Add cooked vegetables with their liquid and puree until smooth. (Or force the cooked vegetables through a sieve or food mill and beat in the skim milk powder and water with an egg beater.) Return to saucepan and stir in salmon, salt, paprika and pepper. Heat just to serving temperature, do not boil after adding the milk.

TO MICROWAVE: Cut margarine in quarters and place in a 1½-quart casserole with onion and celery. Cover and microwave for 3 minutes on full power. Stir in chopped potato and ¾ cup of water. Cover and microwave for 10 minutes on full power. Let stand 2 minutes.

Pour the remaining cup of water into the container of an electric blender, add skim milk powder and blend on high speed for 10 seconds. Add cooked vegetables with their liquid and puree until smooth. (Or force the cooked vegetables through a sieve or food mill and beat in the skim milk powder and water with an egg beater.) Return to casserole and stir in salmon, salt, paprika and pepper. Microwave just to serving temperature—3 to 4 minutes—stirring once. Do not boil after adding the milk.

SUPER-NUTRITION VARIATION:

● Add 2 tablespoons chopped, canned pimiento when pure-eing the other vegetables.

● Add ⅛ teaspoon C-TRATE and the contents of one DAILY B-COMPLEX capsule with the paprika.

Yield: Approximately 5 cups = 4 servings

VITAMIN "P" SOUP

Smooth and rich tasting, amazingly high in protein, vitamins and minerals: one serving of this soup can provide a well balanced and satisfying lunch, even without a salad or sandwich. (Metric measurements are included for convenience when using a scale and a food processor.)

1 tablespoon COLD PRESSED ALL BLEND OIL

2 cups chopped lettuce (150 grams)

1 large carrot (100 grams) peeled or scraped and chopped

1 medium onion (100 grams) chopped

½ large green bell pepper (50 grams) chopped

1 rib celery with leaves (50 grams) chopped

2 tablespoons SOY FLOUR

½ teaspoon SEA SALT

2½ cups beef broth (homemade or canned)

⅔ cup dried split peas (150 grams)

½ of one bay leaf

1 cup water

¼ cup snipped parsley

½ cup non-instant SKIM MILK POWDER

Heat oil in a 3-quart saucepan and stir in lettuce, carrot, onion, bell pepper and celery. Cook and stir for 2 or 3 minutes, but do not brown. Stir in soy flour, salt and beef broth. Cover and bring to boiling over medium heat. Rinse dried peas and add slowly so that boiling does not stop. Add bay leaf, reduce heat and simmer, covered, for 1½ hours—or until vegetables are tender—stirring occasionally.

TO MICROWAVE: Combine chopped fresh vegetables with oil in a 3-quart casserole. Cover and microwave on full power for 3 minutes. Stir in soy flour

22

and salt. Rinse dried peas and stir in with broth. Add bay leaf, cover and microwave for 25 minutes on full power, stirring once. Let stand 5 minutes and test for doneness—if vegetables are not tender, microwave for an additional few minutes.

Ladle soup into the container of an electric blender. Blend on the highest speed until smooth and return to the cooking pan or dish. Pour the cup of water into the blender, add parsley and skim milk powder and blend on high speed. (Or force mixture through a sieve or food mill and beat in skim milk powder, water and parsley with an egg beater.) Stir into the soup and heat just to serving temperature—do not boil after adding the milk. Taste and add freshly ground black pepper and additional salt, if desired.

SUPER-NUTRITION VARIATION:

- Blend with the hot soup: 1 tablespoon LIQUID LECITHIN
  1 tablespoon BREWER'S YEAST
  ½ teaspoon KELP SEASONING
  ⅛ teaspoon C-TRATE

Yield: 6 one-cup servings

WITH SLOW-COOKER: For a 3½- to 4-quart slow-cooker, double all of the ingredients. Combine the lettuce, carrot, onion, bell pepper and celery in the slow-cooker. Stir in oil, rinsed dried peas, broth and salt. Add bay leaf, cover and cook on Low for 8 to 10 hours, until vegetables are tender. Blend the soy flour with the cooked soup, skim milk powder, fresh parsley and water, working in installments and transferring the blended mixture to a large mixing bowl. Freeze portions not needed immediately and heat only the soup to be served.

Yield: 12 one-cup servings

CHAPTER 2

Salads & Dressings

Tossed salads are a delightfully simple way to incorporate enzymes as well as vitamins in the menu. Varying the greens by using spinach, escarole or endive as a change from the various forms of lettuce will avoid monotony. Including shreds of unexpected vegetables (such as Chinese radish, jikima, rutabaga or turnip) adds sparkle. If the accompanying meal is light in protein, bits of cooked meat, poultry or shellfish may be added along with grated cheese and/or chopped, hard-cooked egg. Yogurt and cheese dressings add protein plus calcium, and even "Almost Mayonnaise" has respectable amounts of both (recipes follow).

For a super-nutritional dressing that requires no recipe, simply toss the salad with a spoonful or two of WHEAT-GERM OIL, then add a teaspoon of water in which ⅛ to ¼ teaspoon of C-TRATE has been dissolved. Sprinkle with SEA SALT and freshly ground black pepper and serve while crisply glistening.

ALMOST MAYONNAISE

This easily-prepared milk-mayonnaise contains none of the chemical additives and less than one-third the calories of commercial mayonnaise. (See comparison chart following the recipe.) It will keep in the refrigerator for several weeks and makes a nutritious addition to salads or sandwiches.

⅓ cup non-instant SKIM MILK POWDER
1 tablespoon ARROWROOT (or cornstarch)
1 teaspoon FRUCTOSE GRANULES

¾ teaspoon SEA SALT
½ teaspoon dry mustard powder
¼ teaspoon B-COMPLEX YEAST POWDER
⅛ teaspoon natural celery salt

¹⁄₁₆ teaspoon ground white pepper
¾ cup water
1 large egg
2 tablespoons APPLE CIDER VINEGAR

2 teaspoons fresh lemon juice
2 tablespoons COLD PRESSED SAFFLOWER OIL
1 tablespoon LIQUID LECITHIN
¼ teaspoon C-TRATE

A double boiler may be used for this, but with frequent stirring a single saucepan does very well, and cuts kitchen time. Combine all dry ingredients, except the vitamin C powder, in a saucepan. Gradually add water, stirring to keep smooth. Whisk in egg, then vinegar and lemon juice. Cook and stir over low heat until thickened and beginning to bubble—about 10 minutes. Whisk in oil, lecithin and C-Trate.

> **TO MICROWAVE:** In a 4-cup glass measure, combine dry milk, arrowroot, fructose, salt, mustard, B-complex powder, celery salt and pepper. Gradually add water, stirring to keep smooth. Whisk in egg, then vinegar and lemon juice. Microwave, uncovered, for about 4 minutes on full power—stirring once each minute until beginning to bubble and thicken. Whisk in oil, lecithin and C-Trate.

NOTE: For even smoother mayonnaise: blend oil, lecithin and C-Trate into the hot mixture with an electric blender or food processor. — **Yield: Approximately 1⅓ cups**

COMPARISON CHART

per tablespoon:	Almost Mayonnaise	Commercial Mayonnaise*	Commercial Mayonnaise-Type Salad Dressing*
Calories	31	100	65
Protein	1.04 grams	.10 grams	trace
Fats	.92 g	11.00 g	6.00 grams
Carbohydrates	1.90 g	.30 g	2.00 g
Calcium	28.00 mg	3.00 mg	2.00 mg
Iron	.78 mg	.10 mg	trace
Potassium	39.95 mg	5.00 mg	1.00 mg

*from *The Dieter's Companion*, Nikki & David Goldbeck, Signet, 1977 and *Nutrition Almanac*, McGraw-Hill Paperbacks, 1975.

BLEU CHEESE-SOUR CREAM DRESSING

Combining yogurt with the sour cream reduces the fat calories and adds some beneficial acidophilus in an unidentifiable guise.

⅓ cup sour cream
⅓ cup ACIDOPHILUS YOGURT
1 ounce bleu cheese

Blend yogurt with sour cream, then stir in crumbled cheese. Store in the refrigerator until ready to serve—will keep for several days.

Yield: ¾ cup

COTTAGE CHEESE SALAD DRESSING OR SANDWICH SPREAD

No eggs are needed for this mayonnaise-type salad dressing. Substituting low-fat cottage cheese and skim milk reduces both the calories and fat without altering the sinfully rich texture. (Calories would be lowered from 23 to 18 per tablespoon, and fat from 1.8 grams to 1.1.) Using this dressing for potato salad is a delicious way to turn the salad into a high-protein entree, and the sandwich spread adds nourishment to meals-on-the-run.

½ cup creamed, small-curd cottage cheese (or homemade cottage cheese from the recipe on page 00)
2 tablespoons light cream or milk
1 tablespoon LIQUID LECITHIN
½ teaspoon fresh lemon juice
⅛ teaspoon VITAMIN C POWDER (C-TRATE)
⅛ teaspoon natural celery salt
⅛ teaspoon natural onion salt

Place all ingredients in blender container or food processor bowl and blend until smooth. (Or press the cottage cheese through a sieve and blend with remaining ingredients.) Use in place of mayonnaise for salads or sandwiches. May be thinned with water or milk and additional seasonings added for cole slaw or tossed salads.

Yield: 11 tablespoons

SANDWICH SPREAD:

- Add 2 tablespoons chopped olives, green or ripe
     1 tablespoon pickle relish
     1 tablespoon chili sauce

SUPER-NUTRITION VARIATION:

- Add, if desired: ¼ teaspoon B-COMPLEX POWDER
                   ⅛ teaspoon additional C-TRATE
                   contents of one 5,000 IU SUPER DRY A &
                   D capsule

Yield: 1 cup

TROPICAL SALAD DRESSING OR SAUCE

A spicy, fat-free, sweet-and-sour dressing that does great things for vegetable salads or stir-fry mixtures.

¼ cup firmly packed RAW BROWN SUGAR

1 tablespoon ARROWROOT or cornstarch

½ teaspoon SEA SALT

½ teaspoon ground ginger

¼ teaspoon *each* dry mustard and onion powder

⅛ teaspoon *each* ground black pepper and garlic powder

¼ cup APPLE CIDER VINEGAR

1 cup hot tap water

Mix sugar, arrowroot, salt, ginger, mustard, onion powder, pepper and garlic in a small saucepan. Stir in vinegar, then hot water. Cook and stir over low heat until clear and slightly thickened.

TO MICROWAVE: Combine dry ingredients in a 4-cup glass measure. Stir in vinegar and hot water. Microwave, uncovered, on full power for 4 minutes—or until clear and thickened—stirring each minute.

Store in a covered jar in the refrigerator. Shake before using.

Yield: 1⅓ cups

BEAN SALAD WITH LENTILS

When your freezer is well stocked with a variety of legumes, this salad can be quickly assembled to add delicious nutrition to mealtimes during any season of the year. Ideal for busy-day schedules, pot-luck dinners, or company meals, the flavor improves after spending a day or so in the refrigerator. For a salad luncheon, garnish with olives, wedges of tomatoes and hard-cooked eggs on a bed of crisp greens and accompany with warm rolls.

DRESSING:

2 tablespoons TURBINADO SUGAR
2 tablespoons FRUCTOSE GRANULES
½ teaspoon KELP SEASONING
¼ teaspoon SEA SALT
¼ teaspoon freshly ground black pepper
¼ teaspoon C-TRATE
contents of one 10,000 IU SUPER DRY VITAMIN A & D capsule
¼ cup APPLE CIDER VINEGAR
1 tablespoon water

SALAD:

1 cup drained, cooked, cut green beans
1 cup drained, cooked GARBANZOS (cooking directions for dried legumes are on page 00)
1 cup drained, cooked kidney beans
1 cup drained, cooked LENTILS
1 tablespoon WHEAT GERM OIL
½ cup finely chopped celery
½ cup thinly sliced green onions with crisp tops

Combine the dry ingredients for the dressing in a small saucepan. Stir in vinegar and water and heat until fully boiling. (Or combine in a 2-cup glass measure and microwave for 1 minute.) Let stand, covered.

Place green beans, garbanzos, kidney beans and lentils in a serving dish or refrigerator container and toss with the oil. Stir in celery, onions and dressing. Cover and chill before serving.

VARIATIONS: Red, black, brown or white beans may be substituted for the kidney beans and chopped onion used in place of the sliced green onions. The vitamin A capsule may be omitted, but this is a wonderful opportunity to include a little extra "A" since the vitamin E in the wheat germ oil is there to protect it.   **Yield: 6 servings**

CHICKEN SALAD SUPREME

Grapes provide the touch of elegance for this salad which can double as filling for pocket breads. (Fresh grapes can be washed, blotted dry and quick-frozen on cookie sheets, then stored in a plastic bag in the freezer. Slice while still frozen and serve before they have fully defrosted.)

2 tablespoons ACIDOPHILUS YOGURT	½ cup thinly sliced celery (1 large rib)
2 tablespoons Almost Mayonnaise (recipe on page 27)	1 cup diced, cooked chicken
⅛ teaspoon seasoned salt	½ cup sliced seedless green grapes

Blend yogurt with mayonnaise and salt in a mixing bowl. Cut celery rib in half, lengthwise, before thinly slicing on the diagonal. Add to mixing bowl and toss with chicken to combine. Add grapes just before serving if the salad is prepared ahead and refrigerated. Dust with paprika before serving on crisp greens.

SUPER-NUTRITION VARIATION:

- ½ teaspoon KELP
  contents of one DAILY B-COMPLEX CAPSULE

Yield: 4 servings

COLE SLAW MOUSSE

A wonderfully convenient and nutritious salad that avoids last-minute hustle and cleverly conceals the yogurt with its piquant, garden-fresh flavor.

¾ cup chicken broth (homemade or canned) divided	2 tablespoons Almost Mayonnaise (recipe on page 27)
1 tablespoon unflavored PURE GELATIN	1 teaspoon RAW HONEY
¾ teaspoon seasoned salt	1 teaspoon prepared horseradish
	⅔ cup ACIDOPHILUS YOGURT

1 cup finely shredded cabbage
(4 ounces)

½ cup shredded carrot (2 ounces)

2 green onions with crisp tops, minced

2 tablespoons finely chopped green bell pepper

¼ teaspoon C-TRATE

Heat ½ cup of the broth to boiling. Combine gelatin and salt in mixing bowl. Pour in boiling broth and stir until gelatin is dissolved. Add the remaining ¼ cup of cold broth and stir in with mayonnaise, honey and horseradish. Blend yogurt into the mixture and chill in the refrigerator or freezer.

> **WITH FOOD PROCESSOR:** Place yogurt, mayonnaise, honey and horseradish in processor work bowl with steel cutting blade and process to blend. Add ¼ cup cold broth while the processor is running.
>
> Combine gelatin and salt in a mixing bowl. Heat the remaining half-cup of broth to boiling and stir into gelatin mixture. Add to running processor through the feed tube, then return to the mixing bowl and chill in the refrigerator or freezer while preparing vegetables in the processor.

As soon as the gelatin is syrupy, stir in the vegetables and C-Trate. Transfer to four individual molds or a 3-cup loaf pan. Refrigerate for several hours before serving.

Yield: 4 servings

COLE SLAW WITH HORSERADISH DRESSING

In addition to a full complement of the familiar vitamins and minerals, fresh, raw cabbage contains vitamin U which tests have shown to be both a cure and a preventative of stomach ulcers.*

---

*How to Get Well, Airola, Health Plus, Phoenix, AZ, 1974.
Supernutrition, Passwater, Pocket Books, New York, 1975.

2 tablespoons ACIDOPHILUS YOGURT	⅛ teaspoon freshly ground black pepper
2 tablespoons milk	⅛ teaspoon C-TRATE
2 teaspoons prepared horseradish	2 cups freshly shredded cabbage (5 ounces)
½ teaspoon KELP SEASONING	⅛ teaspoon paprika
¼ teaspoon SEA SALT	

Blend yogurt, milk, horseradish, kelp, salt, pepper and C-Trate. Toss with cabbage, garnish with a sprinkling of paprika and serve at once to retain the full nutritional value of the cabbage.

SUPER-NUTRITION VARIATION:

● Add the contents of 1 DAILY B-COMPLEX and one 5,000 IU SUPER-DRY A & D capsule.

Yield: 4 servings

CURRIED LOBSTER SALAD

Give the lobster solo billing and it may not be necessary to mention that half of that lobster is actually chicken! The nutritional advantages of this salad needn't be mentioned either, just enjoyed along with the great taste. (Metric weights are included for convenience when using a kitchen scale and a food processor.)

½ teaspoon SEA SALT	1 8-ounce can juice-pack crushed pineapple, drained and liquid reserved
½ teaspoon paprika	
½ teaspoon curry powder (more to taste)	
¼ teaspoon C-TRATE	1½ cups cooked BROWN RICE, cooled
¼ teaspoon B-COMPLEX YEAST POWDER	1 cup thinly sliced celery (100 grams)
¼ cup ACIDOPHILUS YOGURT	¾ cup diced, cooked chicken breast
¼ cup Almost Mayonnaise (recipe on page 27)	¾ cup diced, cooked lobster
2 tablespoons natural CASHEW BUTTER	½ cup coarsely chopped cashew nuts (50 grams)
	¼ cup thinly sliced green onions with crisp tops (40 grams)

In mixing bowl combine salt, paprika, curry powder, C-Trate, and B-complex powder. Blend in yogurt, mayonnaise and cashew butter plus 2 tablespoons of the juice drained from the pineapple. Stir in remaining ingredients and chill in a covered container. Serve on a bed of greens and garnish with green olives and tomato wedges.

VARIATIONS:

● When fresh pears are in season, core and dice one large pear in place of the drained pineapple.
● If the food budget requires pampering, forego the lobster and use 1½ cups of diced chicken.

EGGPLANT ANTIPASTO

Similar to Sicilian "Caponata," this entrancing vegetable melange proffers its vitamins and minerals in true Italian style. Serve in a clear glass bowl as an appetizer or a dinner relish; or spoon over greens on individual salad plates and garnish with wedges of hard-cooked egg, rolled anchovies, whole green olives, marinated shrimp or tuna chunks. The eggplant mixture will keep in the refrigerator for over a week and can change nationality when accompanying meat or cheese as a filling for Syrian Pocket Breads. (recipes on pages 181-184)

2 small carrots, peeled or scraped and cut in ¼-inch diagonal slices
1 tablespoon Marsala, cream sherry, or apple juice
1 tablespoon water
¼ teaspoon C-TRATE
2 tablespoons COLD PRESSED VIRGIN OLIVE OIL
½ pound (1 small) eggplant, washed and cut in ½-inch cubes
2 medium ribs celery, cut in ¼-inch diagonal slices
½ medium onion in ¼-inch slices, quartered and the rings separated to make slivers
½ large green bell pepper, slivered

1 tablespoon APPLE CIDER VINEGAR
2 teaspoons FRUCTOSE GRANULES
¾ teaspoon SEA SALT
½ teaspoon KELP SEASONING
½ teaspoon paprika
⅛ teaspoon ground black pepper
⅛ garlic powder
1 cup diced raw, ripe tomato
1 tablespoon capers, drained but not rinsed
¼ cup drained, sliced black olives
1 tablespoon pignolias (pine nuts) (optional)

Combine carrots with wine, water and C-Trate in a skillet. Cover and cook over medium heat until the liquid evaporates—about 5 minutes. Stir in 1 tablespoon oil and the eggplant cubes. Cover and steam until eggplant is heated, then uncover and stir-fry until carrots are tender-crisp and eggplant is translucent. Transfer to refrigerator container or serving dish.

Stir remaining oil with celery, onion and green pepper in the warm skillet. Cover and steam for 3 or 4 minutes, then uncover and stir-fry until vegetables are tender-crisp but not browned. Add vinegar, fructose, salt, kelp, paprika, black pepper and garlic. Stir in with tomato and capers. Cover and bring to a full boil over medium heat. Stir in olives and pignolias (if used) with reserved carrots and eggplant.

> **TO MICROWAVE:** A microwave oven saves calories as well as time and energy by requiring only 1 tablespoon of oil and little stirring—so the vegetables may be prepared in installments while microwaves take care of the stir-frying.
>
> Combine the wine, water, C-Trate and carrots in a 1½-quart casserole. Cover and microwave on full power for 4 minutes. Stir in eggplant cubes, cover and microwave on full power for 5 minutes—stirring after 3 minutes. Transfer to serving dish or storage container.
>
> Combine celery, onions and green pepper with 1 tablespoon of oil in the warm casserole. Cover and microwave for 2 minutes on full power. Add vinegar, fructose, kelp, salt, black pepper and garlic. Stir in with tomatoes and capers. Cover and microwave on full power for 3 minutes. Stir in olives and pignolias, if used, with reserved carrots and eggplant.

Transfer to serving dish or storage container. May be served chilled or at room temperature.

Yield: 3½ cups = 8 servings

Emergency Ration

ONION RELISH-SALAD

The onion rates top billing for this multi-purpose, vitamin-packed vegetable combination as its crisp shreds are most apparent. (Discretion is often the better route to good nutrition and there is no need to mention the zucchini since it is so well camouflaged!) Once you discover the deliciously crunchy-smooth zest this easily-prepared relish adds to any meal, you may want to double the recipe in order to keep a jar in the refrigerator. Serve "as is" for a relish-salad with hot or cold entrees. . . . combine with cottage cheese or yogurt and serve on greens as a luncheon salad. . . . spoon into pocket breads and accompany with sharp cheddar and thin slices of meat loaf for hearty sandwiches or snacks. . . . use as the base for a three-bean salad by combining with cooked kidney beans, garbanzos and green beans. . . . or add to leftover, cooked vegetables with a spoonful of mayonnaise and Swiss cheese cubes for an emergency salad. . . . The possibilities are practically endless, and the relish may be made in quantity for freezing during zucchini season.

2 tablespoons TURBINADO SUGAR	½ cup shredded raw carrot (2 ounces)
¾ teaspoon SEA SALT, divided	¾ pound zucchini (2 cups shredded)
½ teaspoon KELP SEASONING	
⅛ teaspoon ground white pepper	2 medium onions
2 tablespoons APPLE CIDER VINEGAR	1 large green bell pepper, shredded
1 tablespoon water	

Combine sugar, ¼ teaspoon of the salt, kelp and white pepper in a 2-quart saucepan. Stir in vinegar, water and carrot. Cover and bring to a full boil for 1 minute. Let stand. (To microwave: combine in a 2-quart cooking dish, cover and microwave for 3 minutes on full power.)

Scrub zucchini and remove stem ends, but do not peel before shredding. Sprinkle with the remaining half-teaspoon salt and let stand for 10 minutes. Drain in a sieve, pressing gently to squeeze out the moisture. (Reserve this liquid for making soups or stocks.) Quarter onions and slice in a food processor to make shreds or thinly slice and cut each slice in quarters. Remove stem and core from pepper but leave the seeds and shred by hand or with a food processor.

Add zucchini, onion and pepper to the carrot mixture and blend. Transfer to a glass jar or serving dish, cover and store in the refrigerator. The relish may be served immediately, but it improves in flavor after standing and will keep for a week in the refrigerator.

SUPER-NUTRITION VARIATION:

- Stir into the relish: ¼ teaspoon C-TRATE
  contents of one 10,000 IU SUPER DRY A & D capsule

Yield: 2½ cups = 8 relish servings

PEAR-CRABMEAT SALAD

Combine fresh pears with crabmeat, bleu cheese and walnuts for a refreshingly light luncheon salad well supplied with complete protein.

1½ cups diced fresh pears (2 large)
⅛ teaspoon C-TRATE
⅔ cup thinly sliced celery
⅓ cup coarsely chopped walnuts

1 cup (1 6-ounce package frozen) lump crabmeat
3 tablespoons ACIDOPHILUS YOGURT
¼ cup (1-ounce) crumbled bleu cheese

Wash pears, quarter and core; peel only if skin is tough. Cut in ½-inch cubes and toss with the vitamin C powder. Cut trimmed celery ribs in half, lengthwise, and thinly slice on the diagonal. Add to pears with walnuts and crabmeat. Blend yogurt with bleu cheese, adding a little milk if needed, and fold into salad. Serve on a bed of greens.

For a dinner salad, omit the crabmeat and prepare as directed.

Yield: 4 servings

BASIC POTATO SALAD

Everyone has a favorite formula for potato salad, and as with vegetable soup, the more varied the ingredients, the better the flavor. The following recipe is a basic pattern to which may be added sliced radishes, shredded cucumber or zucchini, green or ripe olives, mustard seed, black pepper, etc. Using homemade mayonnaise, an assortment of vegetables, and at least some of the supplements will assure a full range of the necessary nutrients. The protein-carbohydrate ratio is impressive and calories and fats are reduced as shown by the comparison chart.

1¼ pounds potatoes, cooked in their jackets, peeled and sliced to make 4 cups
2 large ribs celery (½ pound)
½ medium onion
½ large green bell pepper
2 tablespoons chopped pimiento
1 tablespoon fresh parsley

4 large eggs, hard cooked
1 cup Almost Mayonnaise (recipe on page 27)
1 teaspoon prepared mustard
¾ teaspoon VEGE-SAL
¼ teaspoon natural celery salt
¼ teaspoon paprika

Chop celery, onion and bell pepper by hand or in a food processor. Add to the sliced potatoes in a 2-quart mixing-serving bowl with the pimiento and parsley. Shell the eggs if necessary (microwaving the eggs in covered custard cups avoids this chore). Chop by hand or in the food processor and blend in with the mayonnaise and mustard. Sprinkle with Vege-Sal and celery salt. Stir, smooth top, sprinkle with paprika and chill before serving.

SUPER-NUTRITION VARIATION:

● Blend ¼ cup ACIDOPHILUS YOGURT and ¼ teaspoon

DOLOMITE POWDER with the mayonnaise

● Add ⅛ teaspoon C-TRATE plus the contents of 1 DAILY B COMPLEX and one 5,000 IU SUPER DRY A & D capsule with the Vege-Sal

Yield: 6 cups = 6 generous servings

COMPARISON CHART

	Basic Potato Salad	Super-Nutrition Variation	Commercial Potato Salad*
per cup of Potato Salad			
Calories	207	213	349
Protein grams	9.48	10.43	7.2
Fat grams	6.50	6.50	22.0
Carbohydrate grams	21.70	22.40	32.3
Calcium milligrams	117.00	176.00	45.8

TROPICAL GARBANZO SALAD

An interesting change-of-pace salad to serve on additional greens as the stellar attraction for a salad luncheon; or to complement a bland pasta entree, a Delicatessen-Style Chicken (recipe on page 100) or a cold meat platter for dinner.

1¼ cups cooked, drained GAR-BANZOS (cooking instructions are on page 123)
1 teaspoon WHEAT GERM OIL
1 cup diced mango (or fresh peach)
¼ teaspoon C-TRATE
¼ teaspoon ground ginger

½ cup minced celery
¼ cup minced green bell pepper
½ cup Tropical Dressing (recipe on page 30)
1 cup finely chopped lettuce, packed
¼ cup COCONUT MEAL

Toss garbanzos with the oil in a mixing bowl. Cut the peeled and seeded mango in cubes the same size as the

---

*Nutrition Almanac, McGraw-Hill, 1975.

garbanzos. Add to the mixing bowl and sprinkle with
vitamin C powder and ginger. Stir in celery, green pepper
and dressing. Cover and refrigerate. Toss with lettuce and
coconut just before serving.

SUPER-NUTRITION VARIATION:

● Add the contents of one DAILY B COMPLEX capsule
with the C-Trate and ginger
● Add 2 tablespoons LECITHIN GRANULES with the lettuce and coconut meal

Yield: 4 servings

Emergency Ration

TUNA SALAD OR SANDWICH FILLING

*Expand the tuna from one small can to provide four nourishing
servings. Serve the salad on a bed of greens; use it to stuff
tomatoes for a light luncheon; or make it into sandwiches and
accompany with bowls of soup for a quick, substantial meal.*

6 tablespoons Almost Mayonnaise (recipe on page 27)	2 medium sized green onions with crisp tops, thinly sliced
¼ teaspoon B-COMPLEX POWDER	1 medium rib celery, finely chopped
1 SUPER DRY VITAMIN A & D CAPSULE (10,000 IU)	1 7-ounce can tuna, drained
	1 large egg, hard cooked and chopped

Mix the B-complex, contents of the vitamin A and D
capsule and the C-Trate into the mayonnaise in a small
mixing bowl. Add all other ingredients and mix thoroughly.

FOR TUNA-STUFFED TOMATOES: Remove tops from
4 medium tomatoes. Hollow out with serrated fruit spoon
and invert to drain. Chop firm pulp and stir into tuna
salad. (The seeds and liquid may be reserved for the soup
pot.) Fill tomatoes with tuna mixture, sprinkle with paprika, and serve on crisp lettuce leaves.

FOR TUNA SANDWICHES: Spread 8 slices of lightly toasted Rice-Bran Wheat Bread (recipe on page 196) with 1 teaspoon mayonnaise each. Put sandwiches together with tuna salad and lettuce leaves. Cut into halves or quarters and garnish as desired.

NOTE: Using Cottage Cheese Salad Dressing (recipe on page 29) and water-pack tuna will lower the calories and fat content, and increase the amount of protein per serving.

Yield: 4 servings

VEGETABLE ICES

To create a mealtime sensation, adopt the European custom of serving sherbets as a first course or a palate refresher with the main dish. Call them Italian "Granites" or French "Sorbets"— although these ices have a light and fluffy texture without any of their grainy iciness—and vary the seasonings to match the menu. Use raw vegetables instead of fruits for fewer carbohydrates and a gloriously colorful, refreshingly different source of extra nutrition. (The essential enzymes present in raw foods are destroyed by cooking; and while large quantities of raw egg white may prevent the B vitamin, biotin, from being assimilated, the small amounts in these ices should be harmless and are necessary for the airy quality.) Each recipe makes approximately two and one-half cups (six servings) and may be kept frozen for up to a week without crystallization.

CUCUMBER-DILL ICE

¼ cup TURBINADO SUGAR
1 teaspoon PURE GELATIN
¾ teaspoon SEA SALT
1 teaspoon dill seed
¼ teaspoon dried dill weed (or 1 teaspoon chopped fresh dill)
⅓ cup water

2 tablespoons APPLE CIDER VINEGAR
1 large cucumber (½ pound)
2 small green onions with crisp tops, cut in half-inch sections
¼ teaspoon C-Trate
1 egg white, stiffly beaten

Combine sugar, gelatin, salt and dill in a small saucepan. Stir in water and heat to simmering. (Or mix in a glass measuring cup and microwave for 1 minute on full power.) Stir in vinegar, let stand for 5 minutes and pour into the container of an electric blender. Scrub cucumber, remove ends and blemishes but do not peel. (All of the vitamin A, most of the iron, and two-thirds of the fiber are in the skin.) Cut in chunks and add to the blender with the onions and C-Trate. Liquefy on high speed. (Or grind the vegetables.) Press through a coarse sieve, just fine enough to retain any whole seeds or vegetable chunks, into a shallow metal pan and freeze until slushy.

Place the frosty mixture in a small mixer bowl or food processor and beat or process with a cutting blade until smooth. Fold in the beaten egg white. Transfer to an airtight plastic container and freeze until solid.

Serve in hollowed out sections of cucumber or scoop onto lettuce leaves and garnish with sprigs of fresh dill and/or a thin slice of scored cucumber cut half-way through and twisted to a butterfly shape. For an even more dramatic presentation, surround with thin slices of cucumber and additional dill weed.

VARIATIONS—*CELERY ICE*

- Omit dill seed and dill weed
- Substitute celery salt for sea salt
- Substitute 2 large ribs of celery, including 1 leafy top, for cucumber.
- Trim and cut in 1-inch sections before blending or grinding.

ZUCCHINI-MINT ICE

- Omit dill seed and weed
- Add 1 tablespoon chopped fresh mint to the blender with the onions, or stir 1 teaspoon dried mint into the sugar mixture before heating
- Substitute zucchini for cucumber
- Garnish with a sprig of fresh mint

NOTE: For a more intense green, add 2 tablespoons chopped fresh parsley or spinach to the blender container before liquefying the cucumber, celery, or zucchini.

PIQUANT CARROT ICE

2 tablespoons RAW BROWN SUGAR
1 teaspoon PURE GELATIN
1 teaspoon mustard seed
1 teaspoon SEA SALT
⅛ teaspoon ground turmeric
½ cup water
3 tablespoons RAW HONEY

3 tablespoons APPLE CIDER VINEGAR
2 large carrots (½ pound)
1 large rib celery
3 tablespoons canned, chopped green chiles
¼ teaspoon C-TRATE
1 egg white, stiffly beaten

Combine sugar, gelatin, mustard seed, turmeric and salt in a small saucepan. Stir in water and honey and heat to simmering. (Or mix in a glass measuring cup and microwave for 2 minutes on full power.) Stir in vinegar, let stand for 5 minutes and pour into the container of an electric blender. Scrape or peel carrots and trim celery. Cut into half-inch sections and add to blender with green chiles and C-Trate. Liquefy on high speed and press through a sieve (coarse enough to allow the passage of all but whole seeds and vegetable chunks) into a shallow metal pan for quick freezing. When slushy, turn into a processor or mixer bowl and process with the cutting blade or beat until smooth. Fold in beaten egg white and transfer to an airtight plastic container to freeze until solid. Serve with an ice cream scoop on a bed of greens or in footed sherbet glasses, garnish with thin celery sticks and/or a parsley sprig.

TOMATO ICE

¼ cup TURBINADO SUGAR
1 teaspoon PURE GELATIN
¾ teaspoon SEA SALT
½ teaspoon paprika
⅛ teaspoon ground white pepper

1 teaspoon dried basil
⅓ cup tomato juice
2 tablespoons APPLE CIDER VINEGAR
½ pound ripe tomatoes

1 ¼-inch slice medium onion	1 tablespoon chopped fresh (or 1
2 tablespoons drained, chopped,	teaspoon dried) basil
canned pimiento	¼ teaspoon C-TRATE
	1 egg white, stiffly beaten

Combine sugar, gelatin, salt, paprika, white pepper and dried basil (if used) in a small saucepan. Stir in tomato juice and vinegar and heat to simmering. (Or mix in a glass measuring cup and microwave for 1 minute on full power.) Stir to dissolve gelatin and sugar. Let stand for 5 minutes and pour into the container of an electric blender. Wash and core tomatoes, peeling only if coarse, and chop into the blender. Add onion, pimiento, fresh basil and C-Trate. Liquefy on high speed and pour into a metal pan for quick freezing. When slushy, turn into a processor or mixer bowl and process or beat until smooth. Fold in beaten egg white and transfer to a plastic container to freeze until solid. Serve in hollowed-out tomato cups, on a bed of greens, or in a footed sherbet glass. Garnish with sprigs of fresh basil or parsley.

VARIATION—*COCKTAIL ICE:*

- Add ¼ teaspoon celery salt with the sea salt
- Add to the blender container with the pimiento:
   1 tablespoon fresh lemon juice
   1 tablespoon prepared horseradish
   ¼ teaspoon Tabasco sauce

Serve on lettuce leaves; surround with cooked shrimp, diced lobster or other seafood; garnish with lemon wedges and parsley sprigs.

CHAPTER 3

Cheeses & Dips—
Appetizers and Snacks

YOGURT

The wondrous nutritional benefits of yogurt have been recognized for many years. Since its rise in popularity during the past decade, biochemists have discovered that in addition to encouraging a flourishing crop of intestinal flora to manufacture our B vitamins, the calcium in yogurt is more apt to be absorbed because of the acid content; and recent scientific tests credit yogurt with lowering both cholesterol and blood pressure levels.*

Not all commercial yogurts are made with the vital acidophilus culture, so making your own with one of the GNC acidophilus starters is recommended. Electric yogurt-makers abound and recipes for using it for everything from soup to sherbet are so plentiful they need not be rehashed here. However, for the benefit of those who do not enjoy the crisp, acid tang, yogurt is camouflaged in numerous dishes throughout this book (see index for listing) and this one off-beat method of making yogurt is included.

EMERGENCY YOGURT

Requiring nothing more complex than a quart jar and wide-mouth thermos bottles, this yogurt can be made in a hotel room or while camping. The only pre-planning necessary is to take along a few small cans of evaporated milk and a quart jar filled with sealed plastic sandwich bags containing 1/3 cup non-instant skim milk powder.

Pre-warm two clean, 1-cup, wide-mouth thermos bottles with hot tap water. In the quart jar, combine 1¼ cups almost-hot tap water (between 125 and 130 degrees) with ⅓ cup skim milk powder and shake to blend. Add ⅓ cup

*Gottlieb, *Prevention Magazine*, August 1979.

evaporated milk (½ of 1 small can) and a tablespoon or two of leftover, plain yogurt. Shake or stir, pour into the thermos bottles, cover and let stand overnight. Transfer the yogurt to paper or plastic cups with lids and cool in an ice chest; or simply eat it for breakfast with a piece of fruit. Either way, be sure to reserve at least a tablespoonful for making the next day's yogurt.

ARAB CHEESE

This no-effort yogurt-cheese not only provides the nutritional benefits of yogurt—it offers gourmet-type cheeses for appetizers, sandwiches, or dessert cheeses to accompany fresh fruit. Possibly discovered when the first caravan master neglected to remove the yogurt from its skin container, this cheese offers salvation when we neglect to remove our yogurt until it separates, but may be made with perfectly-textured yogurt as well.

The original Arabian method is simplicity itself: empty 1 pint of yogurt into a cloth bag and let it drip for 24 hours. Mix a little salt with the solid remainder, and there is your Arab Cheese—healthful, but with a pronounced tang. To update and gourmetize the process and results: Line a 2-cup sieve with dampened, doubled cheesecloth. Place it over a 4-cup measure with a pouring lip and empty the pint of yogurt into the sieve. Lift the cheesecloth ends and secure with a twist-tie to make a bag. As the liquid accumulates, pour it into a jar and refrigerate for adding to future batches of yogurt. After approximately 12 hours, transfer the bag to a refrigerator dish and let it continue to drain for another 12 hours to produce 5 to 7 ounces of semi-soft cheese that will stiffen somewhat with further refrigeration. For the plain Arab Cheese, mix with ⅛ teaspoon sea salt and store in a covered container in the refrigerator—or use in any of the following variations for exciting cheeses without even a hint of yogurt. (There is no nutritional analysis for these cheeses because of the variance in the amount of cheese produced. By utilizing the drained liquid you can be assured of full benefits from all of the yogurt.)

ARAB-AMERICAN CHEESE SPREAD

Arab Cheese made from 1 pint of yogurt
½ cup (2 ounces) shredded, sharp natural cheddar cheese
1 teaspoon RAW HONEY
1 teaspoon LIQUID LECITHIN
½ teaspoon paprika
¼ teaspoon dry mustard powder
¼ teaspoon B-COMPLEX YEAST POWDER (optional)
¼ teaspoon seasoned salt
¼ teaspoon Worcestershire Sauce

Blend all ingredients in a food processor or in a mixing bowl. Transfer to a small serving dish or crock and store in the refrigerator.

ARABIAN CARAWAY CHEESE

Arab Cheese made from 1 pint of yogurt
1 cup (4 ounces) shredded Monterey Jack cheese
1 teaspoon LIQUID LECITHIN
½ teaspoon RAW HONEY
⅛ teaspoon SEA SALT
1 teaspoon caraway seeds

Blend all ingredients in a food processor or with a fork in a mixing bowl. Refrigerate for several hours for the flavors to mellow and for the mixture to thicken.

BONUS: *ROQUEFORT-TYPE SALAD DRESSING*

Remove half of the mixture before adding the caraway seeds. Thin with milk until the desired consistency. Add sea salt and black pepper to taste and pour over a bowl of torn greens for a spectacular salad.

ARABIAN BLEU

A delightfully spreadable dessert or snack cheese that combines the flavor of bleu cheese with the goodness of yogurt and saves money as well as calories.

**Arab Cheese made from 1 cup of
  yogurt
2 ounces natural bleu cheese**

Place in a small mixing bowl and let soften at room temperature. Blend thoroughly and pack into a small serving dish. Cover and refrigerate until ready to serve.

ORANGE-BLOSSOM DESSERT CHEESE

**Arab Cheese made from 1 cup of
  yogurt
2 teaspoons ORANGE BLOS-
  SOM HONEY**

**⅛ teaspoon grated orange peel
¹⁄₁₆ teaspoon SEA SALT
¼ teaspoon orange extract (optional)**

Blend until smooth in a small bowl and store in the refrigerator. For an attractive serving dish, scallop the edges of half an orange rind.

QUICK & EASY COTTAGE CHEESE

Using skim milk powder and a rennet tablet can make the manufacture of this soft-curd cottage cheese almost as simple as the original method of leaving milk in a goatskin bag for several days—and much faster. No cooking is necessary and the only equipment required is a candy or microwave thermometer and a piece of cheesecloth. Standing times are also reduced to a minimum so the finished cheese can be ready to eat in less than four hours.

**4 cups 80-85 degree tap water,
  divided
2 cups non-instant SKIM MILK
  POWDER
1 cup buttermilk**

**1 cup hot water (160 degrees)
½ junket-rennet tablet dissolved
  in 1 teaspoon cold water
½ cup milk, buttermilk or cream
¼ teaspoon SEA SALT**

Measure 1½ cups of water in the container of an electric blender and add the skim milk powder. Blend until no lumps remain and pour into a 3-quart casserole or glass mixing bowl. (Or combine the skim milk powder and water with an egg beater.) Blend buttermilk with 1 cup of water and add to casserole. Rinse blender with remaining water and stir in with the hot water until the temperature reaches 85 to 95 degrees. Stir in dissolved junket-rennet, cover and let stand for 1 hour at room temperature.

Cut through the curd with a spatula to make a checkerboard with ½-inch squares, cutting all the way to the bottom with each stroke. Cover and let stand for 1 hour, stirring gently after 30 minutes.

Line a large sieve or colander with dampened cheesecloth and place it over a larger bowl. Pour in the curds and whey and allow to drain for 1 hour—rocking the corners of the cloth occasionally to hasten the process. Pour off and reserve the whey as it accumulates. Break up the curd with a fork to allow the last of the liquid to drain. Turn cheese into a plastic or glass container. (The 3 or 4 cups of whey can be refrigerated or frozen and used for making future batches of cheese.) Add milk or cream, sprinkle with salt and stir with a fork to blend.

Yield: Approximately 1½ pounds cottage cheese

VARIATIONS:

● For a richer, more mellow cheese, heat 1 cup light cream or ½ cup heavy cream plus ½ cup water in place of the 1 cup of hot water, then mix the completed cheese with light cream instead of milk.

● When whey liquid is available, use it in place of water and reduce the amount of buttermilk to ¼ cup or eliminate it entirely.

● For DRY CURD COTTAGE CHEESE, do not add the half-cup of milk or cream. This solid cheese is ideal for use in Italian recipes or for making cheese spreads.

CUCUMBER DIP

Fresh-from-the-garden flavor is a plus for this low-fat, low-carbohydrate dip with its extra calcium and vitamins. Serve with raw vegetables, homemade potato chips or some of the crackers from pages 62-65.

½ cup dry-curd cottage cheese	contents of one 5,000 IU SUPER DRY A & D capsule
1 teaspoon LIQUID LECITHIN	
1 teaspoon minced chives	¼ teaspoon DOLOMITE POW-DER
½ teaspoon SPIKE	
¼ teaspoon crushed, dried basil	⅛ teaspoon C-TRATE
¼ teaspoon KELP SEASONING	½ medium cucumber (3½ ounces)

Combine all ingredients except cucumber in a food processor work bowl or the small bowl of an electric mixer and process or beat until smooth. Scrub cucumber and remove blemishes but do not peel. Shred directly into the cottage cheese mixture and stir to combine. Will hold in the refrigerator for as long as 24 hours, but the cucumber retains more character when served soon after shredding.

Yield: 4 servings of 3 tablespoons each

DESSERT CHEESE

Neufchatel-type cheese can be made from dry-curd cottage cheese, either homemade or commercial, or from regular cottage cheese that has been rinsed and thoroughly drained. The French have beautifully elaborate perforated ceramic cheese molds for making these un-cured soft cheeses, but cheesecloth and a small sieve or plastic tuna drainer work equally well.

HONEY DESSERT CHEESE

¾ cup dry curd (or rinsed and drained) cottage cheese	1 teaspoon RAW HONEY
	1 teaspoon LIQUID LECITHIN
1 tablespoon cream or top milk	⅛ teaspoon SEA SALT

Thoroughly combine all ingredients with a fork or in a processor work bowl. Press into a tuna drainer or a small sieve lined with cheesecloth and placed over a cup or dish. Let drain for 10 minutes, gently pressing from the outside edges several times. Pour out liquid, replace drainer or sieve over cup, cover with a piece of plastic wrap and weight with a can that fits just inside the mold. Place the entire assembly in a plastic bag and refrigerate for 6 to 48 hours. Remove and serve, or wrap cheese in plastic wrap and refrigerate for up to one week.

Yield: 4 to 5 ounces

VARIATION: *MARSALA DESSERT CHEESE*

¾ cup dry curd (or rinsed and drained) cottage cheese

2 teaspoons marsala wine or cream sherry

2 teaspoons RAW HONEY

1 teaspoon LIQUID LECITHIN

⅛ teaspoon SEA SALT

Prepare as for Honey Dessert Cheese

Emergency Ration

CARAWAY CHEESE SPREAD

Practically a supplement itself, this amazingly delicious, cheddar-like spread adds zest to breads, crackers or fresh fruit. And its combination of cottage cheese and soybeans, augmented with additional supplements, assures well-balanced, high-protein nourishment. For a refreshing, colorfully attractive snack tray, spread slices of unpared apples with Caraway Cheese Spread and arrange them in a circle around an assortment of crackers from pages 62-65.

½ cup packed dry curd (or rinsed and drained) cottage cheese

⅓ cup cooked, drained, mashed YELLOW SOYBEANS*

2 tablespoons safflower margarine

1 teaspoon LIQUID LECITHIN

1 teaspoon paprika

½ teaspoon SEA SALT

¼ teaspoon DOLOMITE POWDER

¼ teaspoon B COMPLEX POWDER

contents of one 5,000 IU SUPER DRY A & D capsule

⅛ teaspoon C-TRATE

2 teaspoons caraway seed

In a food processor work bowl or the small bowl of an electric mixer, combine all ingredients except caraway

---

*Soybean pulp reserved from making soymilk (recipe on page 135) may be substituted for the mashed soybeans.

seed. Process or beat until smooth. (Or combine with a fork in a mixing bowl.) Stir in seeds and pack into a serving jar or dish. Will keep at least a week in the refrigerator, so the recipe may be doubled if desired.

Yield: Approximately ¾ cup

SOYBEAN SPREADS AND/OR DIPS

With "nouvelle cuisine" and the trend toward more frequent but lighter meals, the traditional tray of canapés and appetizers is rapidly being phased out as a "before dinner" attraction. The same types of foods, however, are excellent snacks or mini-meals for the new pattern of eating four to six times each day instead of the old standard of "three square meals" daily. Any of these delicious, versatile, high-protein dip-spreads will keep for days when refrigerated in a covered container. Use them to stuff celery sections, to spread on crackers or thinly sliced bread for canapés, to add interest and food value to regular or pocket-bread sandwiches, or thin a bit and serve with an assortment of raw vegetables and crackers for dunking.

CHEDDAR-OLIVE SPREAD OR DIP

1 cup (4 ounces) shredded sharp natural cheddar cheese
⅔ cup cooked, mashed YELLOW SOYBEANS* (recipe on page 132)
¼ cup Almost Mayonnaise (recipe on page 27)
1 tablespoon LIQUID LECITHIN
1 teaspoon paprika

1 5,000 IU SUPER DRY A & D capsule (optional)
1 DAILY B COMPLEX capsule (optional)
⅛ teaspoon C-TRATE
1/16 teaspoon ground red pepper (cayenne)
¼-⅓ cup cooking liquid from soybeans
¼ cup minced pimiento-stuffed green olives

Blend cheese, soybeans, mayonnaise, lecithin, paprika, contents of the A & D and Daily B Complex capsules, vitamin C and red pepper by hand or in a food processor until smooth. Stir in cooking liquid (or add through proc-

56

essor feed tube) until mixture is the desired consistency, then stir in the green olives.

Yield: 1 ⅓ cups

SPICY EGG & OLIVE SPREAD

¾ cup (3 ounces) shredded sharp natural cheddar cheese
⅓ cup cooked, mashed YELLOW SOYBEANS* (recipe on page 132) (65 grams)
1 tablespoon minced onion
1½ teaspoons prepared horseradish
1½ teaspoons prepared hot mustard
1 teaspoon LIQUID LECITHIN
1 teaspoon BLACKSTRAP MOLASSES

1 teaspoon paprika
1 teaspoon VEGETABLE SALAD POWDER
¼ teaspoon B COMPLEX POWDER (optional)
⅛ teaspoon C-TRATE (optional)
1/16 teaspoon ground red pepper (cayenne)
1 hard cooked egg, shelled
3 tablespoons minced ripe olives (40 grams)

Blend all ingredients except egg and olives with an electric mixer or a fork. Finely chop egg and stir in with minced olives.

WITH FOOD PROCESSOR: Cut cheese in half-inch cubes and place in the processor work bowl with chopping blade. Add drained soybeans, one-half of a thin slice of onion, and remaining ingredients except for the egg and olives. Process until smooth, scraping down sides several times. Remove blade and attach shredding disk. Shred in egg and olives. Stir and use as a spread or transfer to a serving dish.

Yield: 1 cup

SPICY EGG & OLIVE DIP: Blend or process ¼ cup milk into the mixture before adding the egg and olives.

Yield: 1¼ cups

½ cup (2 ounces) shredded Swiss cheese

⅓ cup cooked, mashed YELLOW SOYBEANS* (65 grams)

⅓ cup finely chopped walnuts (34 grams)

1 tablespoon safflower margarine

½ teaspoon paprika

contents of 1 DAILY B-COMPLEX capsule (optional)

contents of 1 5,000 IU SUPER DRY A & D capsule (optional)

⅛ teaspoon C-TRATE (optional)

2 teaspoons LIQUID LECITHIN

1 tablespoon TAMARI SOY SAUCE

3-5 tablespoons cooking liquid from soybeans

Blend all ingredients, except cooking liquid, until smooth. Stir in liquid until the desired consistency is reached.

WITH FOOD PROCESSOR: Place shredded or chopped cheese in processor work bowl with soybeans and process until pureed. Add walnuts, margarine, paprika, supplemental vitamins A, B, C & D (if used) and lecithin and process until thoroughly mixed. With processor running normally, add soy sauce and cooking liquid through the feed tube until the desired consistency is obtained.

Yield: Approximately 1 cup spread

---

*Soybean cooking directions are on page 132 or the pulp reserved from making soymilk (recipe on page 135) may be substituted.

GARBANZO-SESAME DIP

An easily prepared, fat-reduced version of Arabian "Hummus bi Tahina" that will spark any appetizer tray or cocktail hour. Serve as a dunk for celery sticks, other raw vegetables, sections of Arabian pocket breads, or any of the crackers from pages 62-65.

½ cup SESAME SEEDS

1 teaspoon SEA SALT*

¼ teaspoon garlic powder*

⅛ teaspoon ground red pepper (cayenne)

1 cup cooked, drained GARBANZOS (cooking directions are on page 123)

1 tablespoon fresh lemon juice

4-6 tablespoons cooking liquid from garbanzos

WITH FOOD PROCESSOR: Place sesame seeds, salt, garlic and red pepper in processor bowl with steel cutting blade. Process to a coarse powder—about 2 minutes—scraping down sides at least once. Add garbanzos and process until mixture gathers into a ball—about 1 minute. Redistribute the mixture, add lemon juice and, with processor running normally, gradually add the cooking liquid through the feed tube until of the desired consistency.

WITH ELECTRIC BLENDER: Place sesame seeds, salt, garlic and red pepper in blender container and grind to a coarse powder, scraping down sides at least once. Add ¼ cup cooking liquid and lemon juice and blend for 5 seconds. Add garbanzos and blend on medium speed—pushing mixture down into the blades several times—and adding more cooking liquid if needed.

Store in a covered container in the refrigerator until serving time.

Yield: 1¼ cups

VARIATION: *POWER-SAVER INSTANT GARBANZO-SESAME DIP*

1 cup cooked, drained GARBAN-
ZOS (recipe on page 123)
⅓ cup sunflower-sesame butter
1 teaspoon SEA SALT*
¼ teaspoon garlic powder*

⅛ teaspoon ground red pepper
(cayenne)
1 tablespoon fresh lemon juice
4-6 tablespoons cooking liquid
from garbanzos

Mash garbanzos in a flat-bottomed bowl with a potato masher or fork. Stir in sunflower-sesame butter, salt, garlic and red pepper. Add lemon juice and cooking liquid until the proper consistency for a dip. (Or place all ingredients except cooking liquid, in a food processor work

---

*This authentically flavored mixture is quite salty and redolent with garlic; reduce both by one half for a milder dip.

bowl, process until smooth, and gradually add cooking liquid through the feed tube.)

SUPER-NUTRITION VARIATION:

● Add with the garlic powder: ¼ teaspoon C-TRATE
contents of one 10,000 IU
SUPER DRY A & D capsule
contents of one DAILY B-
COMPLEX capsule

CHICKEN LIVER PÂTÉ

Even those who don't like liver will enjoy a few nibbles of this delicious spread. It can be served as soon as it has cooled, but the flavors mellow if allowed to chill for 8 to 24 hours.

2 tablespoons safflower margarine	1 teaspoon APPLE CIDER VINEGAR
¼ cup chopped onion	1 teaspoon BLACKSTRAP MOLASSES
1 clove garlic, minced	
2 tablespoons SOY FLOUR	¼ teaspoon dry mustard
¼ pound chicken livers	¼ teaspoon SEA SALT
1 hard-cooked egg, chopped	⅛ teaspoon ground white pepper

Place margarine, onion and garlic in small pan and cook until simmering. Stir in soy flour and chicken livers. Cover and cook over low heat until livers are cooked, stirring several times.

TO MICROWAVE: Place margarine, onion and garlic in small glass serving dish. Microwave, uncovered, for 1 minute on full power. Stir in soy flour and livers. Cover and microwave on full power for 1 minute. Stir, set control on Defrost (half power), cover and microwave for 2 minutes.

Transfer to food processor or blender and puree until smooth. Add all other ingredients and blend, scraping down sides as needed. Pack into small glass bowl, cover and refrigerate.

When ready to serve: place on serving plate (unmold pâté, if desired), garnish with parsley sprigs and surround with crackers or thin slices of homemade bread, quartered. Serve with a bowl of celery and carrot sticks, cherry tomatoes, etc.

SUPER-NUTRITION VARIATION: *This is an ideal before-going-out-to dinner appetizer. Serve with high-fiber bread or crackers and a bowl of crudités, then enjoy your restaurant meal with a good nutritional foundation and a clear conscience.*

- Sauté onion in only 1 tablespoon of margarine
- Add with dry mustard: 1 tablespoon LIQUID LECITHIN
  ½ teaspoon KELP SEASONING
  ¼ teaspoon B-COMPLEX POW-DER
  ¼ teaspoon C-TRATE

> **Yield: approximately 1 cup**
> **8 servings of 2 tablespoons each**

POTATO CHIPS

Crunchier and tastier than commercial potato chips, these bonus treats cost nothing except a bit of fat and some oven heat, require practically no extra effort; and, since much of the vitamin and mineral content of potatoes is close to the surface, they are also a nutritional bonus. Make them up whenever you peel potatoes for other uses, store the chips in a jar or plastic bag in the refrigerator and freshen by placing them under a cold broiler and heating for two or three minutes before serving.

1 teaspoon safflower margarine	Peelings from 1 pound of pota-toes
1 teaspoon COLD PRESSED ALL BLEND OIL	SEA SALT or other seasonings (optional)

Melt margarine with oil in a skillet on the stove or in a glass pie plate in the microwave oven.

Thoroughly scrub potatoes, remove any blemishes and dry before peeling. Cut long strips into 2-inch sections and toss with warm margarine and oil. Spread in a single layer on a baking sheet and bake for 20 minutes in a preheated 400 degree oven. (Potatoes should be crisp and lightly browned, but not scorched.) Serve plain, sprinkle with salt, or experiment with other seasonings if sodium is being reduced. Vege-Sal or crushed dried herbs make interesting flavor variations. If you need more chips than you have peelings, squander an entire, well-scrubbed potato on the project. Cut in half, lengthwise, and thinly slice with a vegetable peeler; then toss with the oil mixture and bake as directed.

CAUTION: *Do not use* peelings from potatoes that have a layer of green next to the peel as this may contain solanine, a dangerous alkaloid. Potato sprouts also are dangerous and should be completely removed.

NUTRITIONAL NOTE: These chips are not included in the Nutritional Analysis tables because of the number of variables involved, but they are a totally natural food with more nutrients and fewer calories than regular, deep-fried potato chips. If they are being served without a dip, ⅛ teaspoon C-TRATE plus the contents of one 5,000 IU SUPER DRY A & D and/or one DAILY B-COMPLEX capsule may be sprinkled on with the salt or seasonings.

Emergency Rations

SNACK CRACKERS

Delicious alone, these wholesome, natural crackers can be served with soups or used as any snack cracker. Store in a covered container on the cupboard shelf and, if needed, re-crisp by heating in a moderate oven for a few minutes before serving.

SEED CRACKERS

½ cup STONE GROUND WHOLE WHEAT FLOUR	½ teaspoon natural celery salt
¼ cup unsifted, UNBLEACHED WHITE FLOUR	½ teaspoon celery seeds
1 tablespoon WHEAT GERM	¼ teaspoon SPIKE
1 tablespoon LECITHIN GRANULES	2 tablespoons safflower margarine
1 teaspoon CHIA SEEDS	1 tablespoon COLD PRESSED ALL BLEND OIL
	3 to 4 tablespoons cold water

In mixing bowl, blend all ingredients except margarine, oil and water. Cut in margarine with a fork or pastry blender, then stir in oil and water until mixture can be formed into a ball.

WITH FOOD PROCESSOR: With steel blade in place, process the dry ingredients for 3 on/off turns or pulsations. Add margarine and oil and process to blend. With processor running on normal, add water through feed tube until mixture gathers into a ball.

Divide mixture in half for ease in handling. Roll each half between two sheets of waxed paper until slightly thinner than for piecrust. Peel off top sheet of waxed paper and invert onto an ungreased baking sheet. Remove remaining waxed paper and cut into 1¼-inch squares with a pastry wheel or sharp knife. Repeat with remaining half of the dough, re-rolling any uneven squares. Bake in a preheated 375 degree oven for 9 or 10 minutes.

TO MICROWAVE: Prepare dough as directed but divide into thirds and roll each third between sheets of waxed paper. Remove top sheet of waxed paper and invert onto a microwave baking sheet. Cut into 1¼-inch squares with a pastry wheel or sharp knife. (For even baking, remove the four center squares with a spatula.) Microwave on full power for 3 minutes, turning the baking sheet half-way around after 2 minutes. Let stand for 2 minutes before removing.

SUPER-NUTRITION VARIATION:

- Blend with the dry ingredients: 1 ounce ALL-STAR 95% PROTEIN SUPREME powder

  ¼ teaspoon B-COMPLEX POWDER

  ¼ teaspoon DOLOMITE POWDER

  contents of 1 5,000 IU SUPER DRY A & D capsule

- Add an additional spoonful of water, if needed to form into a ball

Yield: 5½ ounces
Approximately 9 dozen 1-inch crackers

CHEESE CRACKERS

1½ cups (6 ounces) shredded, sharp natural cheddar cheese	1 tablespoon LECITHIN GRANULES
½ cup STONE GROUND WHOLE WHEAT FLOUR	¼ teaspoon SEA SALT
¼ cup unsifted, UNBLEACHED WHITE FLOUR	¼ teaspoon B-COMPLEX YEAST POWDER (optional)
1 tablespoon WHEAT GERM	1 tablespoon safflower margarine
1 tablespoon grated Parmesan cheese	1 tablespoon COLD PRESSED WALNUT OIL
	¼ cup cold water

Shred cheese by hand or in a food processor and set aside. In processor work bowl with steel cutting blade (or in a mixing bowl) blend flours, wheat germ, Parmesan cheese, lecithin and salt. Add shredded cheese, margarine and oil and process or stir with a fork until blended. With processor running, add water through the feed tube until mixture gathers into a ball (or add water 1 tablespoon at a time and stir with a fork until mixture can be formed into a ball.)

Divide mixture in half for ease in handling. Roll one half between two pieces of waxed paper until slightly thinner than for piecrust. Peel off top sheet of waxed paper and invert onto an ungreased baking sheet. Remove remaining waxed paper and cut into 1¼-inch squares with a pastry wheel. Remove any uneven squares and roll with remaining dough. Place on baking sheet and cut. Bake in a preheated 375 degree oven for 10 to 12 minutes. (Conventional baking is recommended as the microwaved crackers tend to be chewy rather than crisp.)

Yield: 9 ounces

CHAPTER 4

Entrees

MEATS
POULTRY
SEA FOOD
VEGETARIAN

GOOD OLD MEATLOAF

This meatloaf has that fondly remembered "back home" taste and texture. Actually, of course, it not only has better flavor and doesn't crumble when chilled and sliced for sandwiches, but it also contains a lot of nutrients lacking in the original variety. This recipe makes two meatloaves, enough for a big company dinner, one family meal plus slices for sandwiches and snacking, or the luxury of having an extra meatloaf in the freezer.

½ cup ROLLED OATS
½ cup grated Parmesan cheese
⅓ cup non-instant SKIM MILK POWDER
¼ cup SOY FLOUR
¼ cup WHEAT GERM
1 tablespoon BREWER'S YEAST
1 teaspoon KELP SEASONING
1 teaspoon SEA SALT
1 teaspoon crushed, dried oregano

½ teaspoon chili powder
½ cup beef broth (homemade or canned)
1 small carrot, peeled or scraped
1 medium onion
½ large green bell pepper with seeds and membrane
1 large egg
1 tablespoon BLACKSTRAP MOLASSES
1¾ pounds lean ground beef

In a large mixing bowl, combine rolled oats, cheese, dry milk, soy flour, wheat germ, brewer's yeast, kelp, salt, oregano and chili powder.

Measure broth in blender container. Cut carrot in chunks; add and blend on high speed until liquified. Cut onion and pepper in chunks and add with egg and molasses. Blend until finely chopped. Pour over dry ingredients and stir to blend. Add meat and mix thoroughly.

Moisten hands with water and shape into two oval loaves. Arrange them at least an inch apart on a broiler pan or any double-bottomed pan so any fat can drip through. Bake in a preheated 350 degree oven for 1 hour, or until done.

TO MICROWAVE: Prepare as directed but shape into two untapered logs with flat ends. Place them two inches apart on a microwave bacon rack, or other cooking dish ridged to allow any fat to drain away from the meat. Microwave on full power until the internal temperature reaches 140 degrees—about 16 minutes—turning dish after 10 minutes.

SUPER-NUTRITION VARIATION: As a mealtime meatloaf, this one is already pretty super—but for sandwiches and emergency rations, any or all of the following supplements may be combined with the dry ingredients.
- 2 tablespoons LECITHIN GRANULES
- ½ teaspoon DOLOMITE POWDER
- 1 teaspoon B-COMPLEX POWDER
- 2 10,000 IU SUPER DRY VITAMIN A & D capsules
- ¼ teaspoon C-TRATE

Yield: 10 servings

SUNFLOWER-MUSHROOM MEATLOAF

Glamorize a meatloaf with mushrooms and sunflower seeds, stretch it with soy granules and rolled oats, and reap the triple reward of flavor, nutrition and economy. For super-sophistication, as well as super-nutrition, top it with Mushroom Ketchup from page 157.

¼ cup SOY GRANULES
½ cup beef broth, homemade or canned
¼ pound fresh mushrooms
6 tablespoons SUNFLOWER SEEDS
½ medium onion
⅓ cup ROLLED OATS
⅓ cup non-instant SKIM MILK POWDER
¾ teaspoon SEA SALT
1 large egg
1 teaspoon BLACKSTRAP MOLASSES
¾ pound lean ground beef

Stir soy granules into broth in a small saucepan and bring to boiling. (Or use a 2-cup glass measure and microwave on full power for 2 minutes.) Cover and let stand for 5 minutes.

Wash mushrooms and roll in paper towel to dry.

Grind sunflower seeds in processor or electric blender and place in mixing bowl. Chop onion by hand or in processor and add to mixing bowl with oats, skim milk powder and salt. Stir to blend. Stir in egg, molasses, and warm soy granules. Shred mushrooms with processor or hand grater and stir in with ground beef.

Pack mixture into a loaf pan and bake in a preheated 350 degree oven for approximately 1 hour, or until done.

> **TO MICROWAVE:** Mix as directed. Pack into a microwave baking ring or glass loaf pan and microwave on full power until the internal temperature reaches 145 degrees. (Approximately 8 minutes for ring, 10 minutes for loaf.) Turn dish after 5 minutes for even cooking. Let stand for 1 minute and turn out on serving plate.

SUPER-NUTRITION VARIATION:

- Use only ½ teaspoon sea salt
- Add with the oats: 2 tablespoons BREWER'S YEAST
  1 teaspoon B-COMPLEX POWDER
  1 teaspoon DOLOMITE POWDER
  ½ teaspoon KELP SEASONING

Yield: 1 pound 10 ounces-6 servings, or 4 servings, plus reserve to chill and slice for sandwiches

BEEF BREAKFAST SAUSAGE

Real sausage flavor with less fat and less cooking; plus a bonus of vitamins, minerals and fiber from the soy-extender and

*the nutritional enhancers. Use in any recipe calling for sausage,
or serve the patties at lunch or dinner as well as breakfast.*

¼ cup chicken broth, homemade
  or canned
2 tablespoons SOY GRANULES*
½ pound lean ground beef
¾ teaspoon SEA SALT

1 teaspoon rubbed sage
¼ teaspoon C-TRATE
¼ teaspoon ground marjoram
⅛ teaspoon ground red pepper,
  optional

Combine broth and soy granules in a small saucepan and
heat to boiling. (Or microwave in a glass measuring cup.)
Cover and let stand for 5 minutes. Combine with all other
ingredients, cover and refrigerate from 1 to 24 hours.

FOR SAUSAGE PATTIES: Shape into half-inch thick
patties and place in a cold skillet over low-medium heat.
Cook until lightly browned, turn and cook until as done as
desired. (Beef does not require the long cooking needed for
pork and will dry out if over-done.)

TO MICROWAVE: Preheat a browning skillet according to the manufacturer's directions for hamburg-
ers. Arrange patties in a single layer, cover with a
paper towel and microwave on full power for 2 minutes. Turn patties and microwave for 2 minutes.

FOR SAUSAGE BALLS: Shape meat mixture into small
balls (½-inch for cocktail nibbles, 1-inch for casseroles)
and place in a cold skillet. Cook over medium heat, turning
frequently, until nicely browned on all sides.

SUPER-NUTRITION VARIATION:

● Add: 1 large egg yolk
        2 tablespoons LECITHIN GRANULES
        1 teaspoon KELP GRANULES
        ¼ teaspoon DOLOMITE POWDER
        contents of 1 5,000 IU SUPER DRY A & D capsule

Yield: 4 servings

---

*⅓ cup soy pulp from making Soymilk (recipe on page 135) may be
substituted for the chicken broth and soy granules.

BEEF SAUSAGE WITH LIMA BEANS

High in protein, iron, potassium and fiber, this robust, satisfying casserole tastes rich without a lot of fat calories. The completed casserole holds well in the refrigerator so it may be prepared the day before serving and reheated in a conventional or microwave oven. Stretch it to a dinner for six by serving a first-course Celery Ice (recipe on page 43) and passing broccoli spears, sliced tomatoes and whole-wheat bread with the casserole. (The nutritional analysis of this meal is listed following the casserole totals.) If desired, garnish the casserole for visual appeal and offer a dessert.

1 recipe Beef Breakfast Sausage (recipe on page 71)
1 tablespoon COLD PRESSED ALL BLEND OIL
1 tablespoon safflower margarine
1 medium onion, quartered and thinly sliced
¼ cup STONE GROUND WHOLE WHEAT FLOUR

1 cup Soymilk (recipe on page 135) OR 4 tablespoons SOY FLOUR plus water to make 1 cup
3 tablespoons non-instant SKIM MILK POWDER
1 teaspoon SPIKE
¾ cup cooking liquid from lima beans
2 cups drained, cooked dry LIMA BEANS (cooking directions are on page 123)

Optional Garnish: 10 Crushed Snack Crackers
(recipes on pages 62-65)
1 tablespoon diced pimiento

Shape Beef Sausage mixture into 24 1-inch balls and place in a cold skillet over medium heat. Cook, stirring frequently, until browned on all sides. Remove to serving casserole with slotted spoon. Add oil and margarine to the drippings and stir in the onion shreds. Sauté until onion is limp but not browned. Remove from heat and stir in flour. Blend Soymilk with skim milk powder and stir in with Spike and cooking liquid. Return to heat and stir until simmering and thickened. Add sausage balls and simmer, covered, for 5 minutes. Stir in lima beans and heat to serving temperature. Pour into serving casserole and garnish if desired.

TO MICROWAVE: Shape Beef Sausage mixture into 24 1-inch balls and place in a 10x10-inch, 2-quart casserole. Cover with a sheet of waxed paper and microwave for 3 minutes on full power. Rearrange sausage balls, cover with waxed paper and microwave for 2 minutes. Transfer meat to a paper towel. Add oil and margarine to the drippings. Stir in onion and microwave on full power for 3 minutes, stirring once. Stir in flour, blended Soymilk and skim milk powder, Spike and bean-cooking liquid. Microwave, uncovered, for 4 minutes on full power, stirring twice. Add sausage balls, cover with lid or plastic wrap and microwave for 3 minutes. Stir in lima beans, cover and microwave for 3 minutes. Let stand for 3 or 4 minutes before serving. Garnish, if desired.

To Prepare Ahead: Prepare as directed but do not heat after adding lima beans. Cover and refrigerate up to 24 hours. Sprinkle with cracker crumbs (if used) and heat to serving temperature in a moderate, conventional oven. (If heating casserole in a microwave oven, microwave for 4 minutes on full power, stir and sprinkle with cracker crumbs, if used, then microwave to serving temperature.) Garnish with pimiento, if desired, just before serving.

SUPER-NUTRITION NOTES:

• If casserole is not to be accompanied by broccoli, carrots, or other vegetables high in vitamin A, add the contents of at least one 10,000 IU SUPER DRY A & D capsule with the Spike.

• If not serving whole wheat bread, add the contents of one DAILY B-COMPLEX capsule with the spike.

Yield: 4 whole-meal servings
6 servings with vegetables and bread

DOUBLE BEAN & BEEF STIR-FRY

With Instant Liquid Tenderizer to turn round steak into tender-
loin, and soybeans for extra protein, half-a-pound of meat can
provide high-protein gourmet-fare for four—and if any of them
are calorie counters, serve shredded lettuce instead of brown rice
as a base for this unusual Oriental dish.

½ pound boneless, trimmed round
steak
¼ teaspoon ground ginger
⅛ teaspoon garlic powder
3 tablespoons TAMARI SOY
SAUCE
1 tablespoon dry sherry or apple
juice
½ teaspoon INSTANT LIQUID
TENDERIZER
⅔ cup beef broth, homemade or
canned

1 10-ounce package frozen cut
green beans, defrosted enough
to separate
1 tablespoon COLD PRESSED
PEANUT OIL
⅓ cup thinly sliced green onions
with crisp tops
1½ tablespoons ARROWROOT
or cornstarch
1 cup drained cooked YELLOW
SOYBEANS (cooking direc-
tions on page 132)
¼ cup sliced water chestnuts

Cut steak into thin strips and marinate in a mixture of
the ginger, garlic, soy sauce, sherry and liquid tenderizer
for 15 minutes.

Bring broth to boiling in a small saucepan and stir in
green beans. Cover and cook for 5 minutes. Remove from
heat and let stand. (The beans will be tender-crisp—for
well-done beans, cook for another 5 minutes.)

Heat oil in a wok or skillet and stir-fry onions until
limp. Lift meat from marinade and stir with the onions
until the pink disappears. Blend arrowroot with the remaining
marinade and stir in with the green beans and their cooking
liquid. Cook and stir for a minute or so, then add soybeans
and water chestnuts. Cook and stir until beans are hot,
then serve over fluffy brown rice or shredded lettuce.

TO MICROWAVE: Cut steak into thin strips and
marinate in a mixture of the ginger, garlic, soy sauce,
sherry and liquid tenderizer for 15 minutes.

Stir green beans into broth in a 4-cup glass measure, cover and microwave on full power for 5 minutes. Let stand. (Beans will be tender-crisp—stir and microwave for 4 more minutes for well-done beans.)

Combine onions with oil in a 1½-quart serving dish-casserole. Cover and microwave on full power for 2 minutes. Lift meat from marinade and stir into onions. Leave uncovered and microwave for 2 minutes on full power. Blend arrowroot with the remaining marinade and stir in with the green beans and their cooking liquid, the soybeans and water chestnuts. Microwave, uncovered, for 4 minutes, stirring once. Serve over fluffy brown rice or shredded lettuce.

SUBSTITUTIONS:
● Cooking liquid from the soybeans may be used in place of any amount of the beef broth
● Thinly sliced celery or chopped bamboo shoots may be substituted for the water chestnuts

SUPER-NUTRITION VARIATION:

● Blend with the arrowroot before stirring in liquid:
  contents of 1 5,000 IU SUPER DRY A & D capsule
  contents of 1 DAILY B-COMPLEX capsule
  ⅛ teaspoon C-TRATE

Yield: 4 servings

DEPRESSION GOULASH

There's nothing depressing about this hearty meal-in-a-dish, but it did originate during the great depression of the thirties and retains its nostalgic, comforting, real-food-in-the-kitchen appeal in spite of substituting steak for hamburger and increasing its nutritional content. It's still a marvelously nourishing and economical stand-by which can be served immediately, refrigerated for several days, or frozen to keep on hand for emergencies. With a salad, rolls, and a fruit dessert, it provides an enjoyable meal for family or guests at any time of year.

3 cups cooked, drained whole-wheat macaroni (1¼ cups dry)

2 tablespoons ACIDOPHILUS YOGURT

¾ pound lean, trimmed, boneless sirloin or round steak, in ¼-inch cubes

INSTANT LIQUID TENDERIZER

1½ cups chopped tomatoes, fresh or canned

2 tablespoons COLD PRESSED ALL BLEND OIL, divided

½ large green bell pepper

1 medium onion, chopped

2 tablespoons WHOLE WHEAT PASTRY FLOUR

2 tablespoons SOY FLOUR

½ teaspoon crushed, dried basil

½ teaspoon SEA SALT

⅛ teaspoon garlic powder

1 small carrot, scraped or peeled and cut in chunks

¼ cup beef broth, homemade or canned

1 teaspoon BLACKSTRAP MOLASSES

6 ounces natural cheddar cheese, chopped

Toss hot macaroni with yogurt in 2-quart casserole. Cover and set aside. Sprinkle meat cubes with tenderizer and let stand.

Chop tomatoes into measuring cup. Heat 1 tablespoon oil in skillet. Chop bell pepper, placing seeds and membrane in the container of an electric blender.

Sauté pepper and onion in the oil until limp but not browned, stirring frequently. Stir in wheat and soy flours, basil, salt and garlic.

Drain liquid from tomatoes into the blender; add carrot chunks and broth. Liquefy on high speed and pour into skillet. Cook and stir until thickened, then add tomatoes and return to boiling. Stir in molasses and add cheese. Cover and let stand to melt the cheese.

In another skillet, heat the remaining tablespoon of oil and saute the beef cubes until well seared and tender, stirring constantly.

If serving immediately: Stir macaroni and meat into the skillet with the sauce and reheat to serving temperature.

If preparing ahead: Combine ingredients in serving or freezing containers and reheat in conventional or microwave oven before serving.

TO MICROWAVE: Prepare macaroni and yogurt,

meat cubes, and tomato as directed. Microwave pepper, onion and oil in 2-quart casserole for 2 minutes on full power. Add flours and seasonings, then stir in blender contents and microwave for 2 minutes. Stir in tomatoes and microwave for 2 minutes. Add cheese, cover and let stand. Microwave meat on a paper plate for 2 minutes on full power, stirring and rearranging after 1 minute. Combine all ingredients in the casserole with the onions and reheat to serving temperature or cool and refrigerate. (To freeze: Transfer to metal or plastic containers without further heating.)

SUPER-NUTRITION VARIATION:

● Add ½ teaspoon KELP SEASONING and ¼ teaspoon B-COMPLEX POWDER with the salt
● Stir in 2 tablespoons LECITHIN GRANULES and ¼ teaspoon C-TRATE with the cooked meat
● Stir in the contents of one 10,000 IU SUPER DRY A & D capsule before reheating to serve

Yield: 6 servings

INSTANT SWISS STEAK

Instant Liquid Tenderizer up-grades the round steak and the vitamin-packed sauce up-grades the nutritional value for a quick and delicious entree.

1½ pounds boneless, trimmed round steak, ¾-inch thick	1 tablespoon PEANUT OIL
INSTANT LIQUID TENDERIZER	½ cup canned tomatoes and liquid
3 tablespoons WHOLE WHEAT PASTRY FLOUR	1 medium carrot
	½ medium onion
2 tablespoons SOY FLOUR	1 teaspoon BLACKSTRAP MOLASSES
1 teaspoon SEA SALT	½ teaspoon KELP SEASONING

WITH 3 or 4-QUART PRESSURE COOKER: Cover meat with tenderizer and pierce with a fork. Cut into 4 serving pieces. Mix flours and salt on a sheet of waxed paper and press into the meat—no need to pound. Heat half the oil in the pressure cooker and sear 2 of the steaks. Remove and sear the last 2 steaks in the remaining oil. Remove steaks and pour ¼ cup water into the pressure cooker. Put in rack and meat. Combine remaining ingredients in the container of an electric blender and blend on high speed until smooth. Pour over steaks. Close cover. Set pressure control for full pressure. When pressure is reached, cook 10 minutes and reduce pressure immediately under running water.

WITH MICROWAVE OVEN: Cover meat with tenderizer and pierce with a fork. Cut into 4 serving pieces. Mix flours and salt on a sheet of waxed paper and press into meat—no need to pound. Preheat microwave browning skillet, add oil and sear steaks for 2 minutes on each side, covering them with a paper towel to prevent splatters. Combine remaining ingredients in blender container and blend on high speed until smooth. Pour over steaks, cover and microwave 5 minutes on full power. Turn steaks, cover and microwave for 3 minutes.

Serve steaks on individual plates with sauce spooned over the top.

SUPER-NUTRITION VARIATION:

● Lift steaks from sauce and place on individual plates. Create your own Lemon-Pepper Flavoring by stirring into the sauce before spooning over meat:

    ¼ teaspoon C-TRATE
    contents of 1 DAILY B-COMPLEX capsule
    ⅛ teaspoon freshly ground black pepper

Yield: 4 servings

BREADED CALVES' LIVER

Even those who don't enjoy restaurant-style liver and onions will relish this tender, quickly cooked variation with its tremendous amounts of iron and vitamins securely encased in a savory coating.

1 pound sliced calves' liver
2 tablespoons evaporated milk
½ cup Seasoned Flour (recipe on page 154)

2 tablespoons COLD PRESSED PEANUT OIL

Rinse liver and pat dry with paper towels. Remove membrane and cut into strips approximately 1x3 inches. Stir with evaporated milk and turn in seasoned flour on a paper towel. Heat oil in skillet over medium heat and sauté liver until lightly browned on both sides but still slightly pink in the center.

TO MICROWAVE: Prepare liver as directed. Preheat browning skillet or grill according to manufacturer's directions. Add oil and liver and microwave for 3 minutes on full power. Turn liver pieces and microwave for another 3 minutes on full power.

Serve with Swiss Potatoes & Onions (recipe on page 118) or sauté sliced onions in another skillet.

Yield: 4 servings

LAMB WITH ARTICHOKE HEARTS

Artichokes are practically synonymous with the word "gourmet" and, when combined with these tenderly flavorful bites of lamb, are truly fare for the discriminating. Trimming all fat from the lamb avoids any hint of the tallow-like, muttony flavor.

¼ cup dry white wine or apple
juice

1 teaspoon TAMARI SOY
SAUCE

¼ teaspoon freshly ground black
pepper

⅛ teaspoon crushed, dried rosemary

⅛ teaspoon garlic powder

1 tablespoon COLD PRESSED
PEANUT OIL

1 pound lean, boneless lamb

½ teaspoon INSTANT LIQUID
TENDERIZER

1 9-ounce package frozen artichoke hearts

½ teaspoon SEA SALT

Combine wine, soy sauce, pepper, rosemary, garlic and
oil in a 1½-quart flame-proof ceramic casserole or glass
bowl. Trim fat and membrane from lamb, cut into 1-inch
pieces and stir into the marinade. Cover and refrigerate for
at least 1, or up to 24 hours.

Remove from refrigerator, stir in tenderizer and let stand
at room temperature for 15 minutes. If a bowl was used for
marinating, transfer to a thick-bottomed skillet or saucepan
and bring to boiling over medium heat. Reduce heat, cover
and simmer until lamb is tender, about 30 minutes, adding
a little water if necessary. Quarter artichoke hearts and stir
in with salt. Cover and simmer 10 minutes.

TO MICROWAVE: Trim and marinate lamb as
directed, using a 1½-quart casserole. Stir in tenderizer and let stand at room temperature for 15 minutes.
Microwave, uncovered, for 2 minutes on full power.
Quarter artichoke hearts and stir in with salt. Cover
and microwave for 5 minutes on full power, stirring
once.

If desired, garnish with fresh parsley or mint leaves
before serving.

SUPER-NUTRITION VARIATION:

● Add with the black pepper: ½ teaspoon KELP SEA-
SONING

- Add with the salt: Contents of 1 5,000 IU SUPER DRY A & D capsule
  ⅛ teaspoon C-TRATE

Yield: 4 servings

ORIENTAL PORK INDOOR BARBECUE

This marinade not only flavors and tenderizes the meat; it imparts a smoky barbecue effect with either a conventional or microwave oven and without any smoky barbecue—and furnishes some extra vitamins as well. Pork loin ribs average twice the meat with half the fat of pork spare ribs—when they aren't available, thick-cut pork loin chops make a delicious substitute.

¼ cup TAMARI SOY SAUCE
¼ cup RAW HONEY
¼ cup Instant Ketchup (recipe on page 156)
¼ cup water
1 teaspoon grated orange peel
1 teaspoon natural "Liquid Smoke"

¼ teaspoon garlic powder
¼ teaspoon C-TRATE
contents of 1 10,000 IU SUPER DRY VITAMIN A & D capsule (optional)
3 pounds pork loin ribs

Combine all ingredients except meat in a glass or plastic container. Turn ribs in the mixture so each is thoroughly coated, cover and refrigerate for 2 to 24 hours. Turn ribs and let stand at room temperature for a few minutes before cooking.

Lift meat from the marinade to a rack over a shallow baking pan and bake in a preheated 325 degree oven for 1 hour. Brush with marinade and turn ribs. Lower heat to 300 degrees and bake for 1½ to 2 hours (until meat is very tender) brushing with marinade and turning at least once more. If any marinade remains, spread it on the ribs 5 minutes before removing from the oven.

TO MICROWAVE: Marinate meat as directed. Lift ribs from marinade to a microwave bacon rack and sprinkle with INSTANT LIQUID TENDERIZER. Let stand 5 minutes. Cover with waxed paper and microwave on full power for 10 minutes, turning dish once. Pour liquid from drip well; brush ribs with marinade, turn and rearrange—placing larger pieces toward the outside. Cover with waxed paper and microwave for 15 minutes on full power, turning ribs and brushing them with the last of the marinade after 8 minutes.

Yield: 6 servings

PORK CHOP PILAF

Pork is higher in B vitamins than other meats and, when the excess fat is removed, is calorically equivalent with beef. This pork chop dinner-in-a-dish is delicious any time of year. Bake it in the oven when the heat will add welcome warmth or use the pressure cooker variation for an easy, substantial meal to provide energy for summer activities without squandering it in the kitchen.

1½ cups chicken broth, home-made or canned
½ cup raw BROWN RICE
½ teaspoon KELP SEASONING
½ teaspoon paprika
¼ teaspoon SEA SALT
¼ teaspoon chili powder

4 large, center-cut pork chops (1½ pounds) trimmed of all solid fat
2 medium onions
1 large green bell pepper
1 cup Mexican Chili-Cheese Sauce (recipe on page 160) or other tomato sauce

Bring broth to boiling in a 2-quart saucepan. Stir in rice, kelp, paprika, salt and chili powder. Cover and simmer for 10 minutes.

While rice is simmering, sear the pork chops in a heavy skillet and set aside. Quarter onions, lengthwise, and thinly slice by hand or in a food processor. Quarter pepper, remove core and seeds and cut pepper into short, quarter-inch-thick slices. Briefly sauté onion and pepper in the drippings left from the pork chops. Transfer to a 2-quart casserole large enough to hold the meat in a single layer.

83

Arrange pork chops over the vegetables and pour in the boiling rice mixture. Cover tightly and bake in a preheated 350 degree oven for 45 minutes to 1 hour, until rice and chops are tender. Serve with heated tomato sauce (recipe on page 159).

WITH 3 or 4-QUART PRESSURE COOKER: Place pork chops in open pressure cooker, sear on both sides over high heat and remove. Quarter onions and thinly slice by hand or in a food processor. Quarter pepper, remove core and seeds and cut pepper into short, quarter-inch-thick slices. Briefly sauté onion and pepper in the drippings. Stir in rice. Add 1 cup broth, kelp, paprika, salt and chili powder. Stir to combine and arrange meat atop. Secure cover and put pressure control in place. Cook for 10 minutes after full pressure is reached. Let pressure go down of its own accord for 5 minutes, then cool under running water. Serve with heated tomato sauce.

SUPER-NUTRITION VARIATION:

● Pour 1 cup of the chicken broth into an electric blender container and add:
  1 small carrot, scraped or peeled and cut in chunks
  Core and seeds from the green bell pepper
  2 tablespoons SOY FLOUR
  ½ teaspoon DOLOMITE POWDER
  ¼ teaspoon B-COMPLEX POWDER
Blend on high speed until the carrot and pepper are liquified, then heat with remaining broth for the oven version, or stir into the pressure cooker as directed.

Yield: 4 servings

GREAT NORTHERN CASSEROLE

Actually a simplified French Cassoulet, this delicious mélange of meat, poultry, beans and vegetables requires only a salad and hot rolls to complete the menu.

½ cup Quick & Easy Tomato Sauce, divided (recipe on page 158)
¼ cup red table wine
1 teaspoon BLACKSTRAP MOLASSES
2 small chicken breasts, split and skinned (1¼ pounds)
1 medium onion, chopped
2 medium ribs celery, chopped
¼ pound extra-lean ground beef
¼ teaspoon rubbed sage
⅛ teaspoon garlic powder
1 tablespoon ARROWROOT or cornstarch
½ teaspoon paprika
½ teaspoon SEA SALT
⅛ teaspoon ground black pepper
1½ cups cooked Great Northern white beans, drained
1 tablespoon snipped parsley

Combine ¼ cup of the tomato sauce with the wine and molasses in a glass or plastic bowl. Turn chicken in marinade, cover and let stand 20 minutes at room temperature, or up to 24 hours in the refrigerator.

Sauté onion and celery with beef in a large skillet, stirring frequently, until vegetables are limp but not browned. Stir in sage, garlic, chicken and marinade. Cover tightly and simmer for about 45 minutes, until chicken is tender, stirring and turning chicken several times.

Combine arrowroot, paprika, salt and pepper with remaining ¼ cup tomato sauce. Stir into simmering mixture. Add beans and parsley. Cover and simmer 5 minutes, stirring occasionally.

TO MICROWAVE: Marinate chicken in tomato sauce, wine and molasses as directed.

Combine ground beef with onion and celery in a 1½-quart casserole. Microwave, uncovered, for 4 minutes on full power, stirring once. Stir in sage, garlic, chicken and marinade. Cover and microwave on full power for 10 minutes. Stir, turn and rearrange chicken, cover and microwave on full power until chicken is tender—about 5 minutes.

Combine arrowroot, paprika, salt and pepper with remaining ¼ cup tomato sauce. Stir into simmering mixture. Add beans and parsley. Microwave, uncovered, until beans are heated through—about 3 minutes on full power.

VARIATION: Substitute 1½ cups cooked dry LIMA BEANS, drained, for the Great Northern white beans.

SUPER-NUTRITION VARIATION:

- Add with the paprika:
  ¼ teaspoon DOLOMITE POWDER
  contents of 1 DAILY B-COMPLEX CAPSULE
  contents of 1 5,000 IU SUPER DRY A & D capsule

Yield: 4 servings

POT AU FEU PLUS BROTH

With a loaf of crusty bread plus some fruit and cheese for dessert you can serve a genuine French repast, including a first-course soup, from this easily prepared, vitamin-packed "boiled dinner."

1 pound lean, boneless round steak, trimmed of visible fat
INSTANT LIQUID TENDERIZER
1 teaspoon SEA SALT
1 cup chicken broth, homemade or canned
1½ cups water
½ cup tomato juice

4 frying-chicken thighs (1 pound) skinned
4 slender carrots (½ pound) scraped or peeled
4 medium potatoes (1 pound) peeled if desired
1 10-ounce package frozen whole green beans, defrosted enough to separate

¼ teaspoon whole peppercorns   1 cup (5 ounces) frozen, small
⅛ teaspoon crushed, dried thyme   boiling onions
1 small bay leaf

Cut steak into 4 serving pieces, sprinkle with tenderizer and let stand 5 minutes. Spread salt in a heavy 3 or 4-quart saucepan and quickly sear meat over high heat.

Stack the steaks on one side of the pan and stir in broth, water and tomato juice. Rearrange meat in a single layer and place the chicken pieces atop. Cut carrots in half, crosswise, and push down in the liquid. Cover with a tight-fitting lid and bring to boiling. Reduce heat and simmer 20 minutes. Gently rearrange the meat and chicken pieces. Cut potatoes in half and add with the green beans, peppercorns, thyme and bay leaf. Cover and simmer for 40 minutes, or until meat and vegetables are tender. Add onions, cover and simmer for 5 minutes.

WITH SLOW-COOKER: Cut steak into 4 serving pieces and place in a 3½- to 4-quart slow-cooker with carrots and potatoes atop. Add chicken thighs, green beans and onions. Sprinkle with salt, thyme and peppercorns. Pour in broth, water and tomato juice. Add bay leaf, cover and cook on Low for 12 hours or until meat and vegetables are tender.

With a slotted spoon, lift out vegetables, chicken and meat. Arrange on a serving platter, cover with foil and/or place in a 200 degree oven to keep warm. Strain broth and pour into small soup cups for serving as a first course.   **Yield: 4 servings**

WITH 4 to 6-QUART PRESSURE COOKER— POT AU FEU FOR 8: Substitute 2 medium onions, coarsely chopped, for the boiling onions and double all other ingredients.

Cut the steak into 8 serving pieces, sprinkle with tenderizer and let stand for 5 minutes. Spread salt in the bottom of the pressure cooker and sear the meat over high heat. Remove steaks and sauté the chopped onion until limp. Stir in chicken broth, water and tomato juice. Add carrots and place the meat atop. Secure cover and bring up to full pressure. Allow to cook for 1 minute and reduce pressure under running water. Add chicken, potatoes, green beans, peppercorns, thyme and 1 large bay leaf. Close cover and bring to full pressure. Cook for 10 minutes, then cool under running water to reduce pressure.

Lift out vegetables, chicken and meat with a slotted spoon and arrange on a serving platter. Cover with foil and/or place in a 200 degree oven to keep warm. Strain broth and pour into small soup cups for serving as a first course.

WITH MICROWAVE OVEN: When time is of the essence, Pot au Feu can be ready to serve to four in less than 30 minutes—with a few alterations in the form of the ingredients and the magic of microwaves.

1 cup beef broth, home-made or canned	INSTANT LIQUID TEN-DERIZER
1 cup chicken broth, home-made or canned	½ teaspoon TAMARI SOY SAUCE
½ cup tomato juice	4 slender carrots (½ pound) scraped or peeled
½ cup water	
1 teaspoon SEA SALT	1 10-ounce package frozen whole green beans, de-frosted enough to sepa-rate
⅛ teaspoon each ground black pepper and crushed, dried thyme	
1 small bay leaf	1 whole chicken breast (1 pound)
1 pound lean, boneless round or sirloin steak, trimmed of visible fat	1 cup (5 ounces) small, fro-zen boiling onions

In a 2-quart casserole, combine beef and chicken broth, tomato juice, water, salt, pepper and thyme. Cover and microwave on full power until boiling—about 7 minutes.

While the liquids are heating, cut steak into ¾-inch cubes. Place in a glass pie plate, sprinkle with tenderizer and soy sauce and toss to cover all sides. Let stand.

Cut carrots into 1-inch diagonal slices and add to the boiling broth. Cover and microwave for 2 minutes. Quarter potatoes and add with green beans. Cover and microwave for 10 minutes on full power—potatoes should be almost tender.

Skin and bone chicken breasts and cut in 1-inch pieces. Stir into boiling broth with onions. Cover and microwave on full power for 2 minutes, or until fully boiling. Remove from oven and let stand.

Cover the plate of steak cubes with a paper towel and microwave for 4 minutes on full power—stirring to rearrange after 2 minutes. Stir into the casserole with the drippings. Pour through a large sieve and remove bay leaf. Spoon the solids back into the casserole, arranging the potatoes on one side with a colorful dividing row of vegetables, then meat and poultry. Cover to retain heat while serving broth as a first course. Reheat the casserole for a minute or so, if necessary.

SUPER-NUTRITION VARIATION: Already super-nutritious, this meal requires very little supplementing; but since natural vitamin C is destroyed by cooking, stirring ⅛ to ¼ teaspoon C-TRATE into the broth after straining will assure an adequate amount, and additional calcium and B vitamins will be supplied by the bread and dessert.

NOTE: For more generous servings of the first-course soup, add 1 or 2 cups of chicken or beef broth to the cooking liquid.

ALFALFA-SPROUT EGG FU YONG

This Americanized version of the Oriental favorite glorifies sprouted alfalfa seeds and supplements the vitamins so that nothing else is needed for a complete meal except a serving of fluffy, hot brown rice and a few slices of ripe tomato with a parsley sprig as a colorful garnish.

3 large eggs
1 teaspoon TAMARI SOY SAUCE
¼ teaspoon ground ginger
¼ teaspoon B-COMPLEX YEAST POWDER
⅛ teaspoon C-TRATE
1 cup coarsely chopped ALFALFA SPROUTS (100 grams)
⅔ cup finely chopped celery (100 grams)

⅓ cup finely chopped green bell pepper (50 grams)
⅓ cup thinly sliced green onions with crisp tops (50 grams)
1 cup finely chopped cooked chicken
2 tablespoons LECITHIN GRANULES
1 tablespoon COLD PRESSED PEANUT OIL (1 teaspoon if using microwaves)

SAUCE:

2 tablespoons ARROWROOT or cornstarch
1 tablespoon cold water

1 cup chicken broth, homemade or canned
1 tablespoon TAMARI SOY SAUCE

Whisk eggs with 1 teaspoon soy sauce, ginger, B-complex powder and C-Trate. Chop vegetables by hand or in a food processor and stir in with the egg mixture, chicken and lecithin granules.

Heat oil in a large skillet and spoon in Fu Yong mixture to make 4 large or 8 small patties. Fold any thin portions of the egg up over the vegetables and turn to brown the reverse sides.

TO MICROWAVE: Oil a microwave omelet cooker with 1 teaspoon of peanut oil and divide Fu Yong mixture evenly into both sides of the pan. Microwave on full power for 4 minutes (until eggs are set and vegetables are tender-crisp) rotating pan one-quarter turn each minute. Cut each half into two pieces to make 4 servings.

SAUCE: Blend arrowroot with water and stir in broth and the tablespoon of soy sauce. Cook and stir over low heat until clear and thickened. (Or mix in the serving dish and microwave, uncovered, for 4 minutes on full power, stirring once each minute.)

Spoon a bit of sauce over the patties and pass the remainder.

SUBSTITUTIONS:

- ⅓ cup chopped water chestnuts may be sutstituted for ⅓ cup of the celery
- 1 cup finely chopped beef or pork may be substituted for the chicken, and beef broth used in place of the chicken broth.

VARIATION: *VEGETARIAN EGG FU YONG*

- Omit chicken and chicken broth
- Add 1 4-ounce can mushrooms, drained and chopped, with the vegetables
- Add ¼ cup PUMPKIN SEED MEAL with the lecithin granules
- Add ¼ teaspoon DOLOMITE POWDER with the lecithin granules
- Use liquid drained from mushrooms plus water to make 1 cup for the sauce

Yield: 4 servings

CHICKEN & BROCCOLI ROYALE

Total gourmet results are equal to more than the sum of the simple ingredients in this dish. The alcohol evaporates from the combination of wines, leaving only the delectable flavor—table wines are best to use for cooking as they are smoother and do not contain the salt added to cooking wines.

10 ounces broccoli spears, cooked
until barely tender

CHICKEN & MARINADE:

1 large chicken breast (1 pound)
1 teaspoon ARROWROOT or
cornstarch

1 teaspoon SESAME OIL
¼ cup Marsala wine or cream
sherry

CREAM SAUCE:

2 tablespoons COLD PRESSED
SAFFLOWER OIL
2 tablespoons safflower margarine
¼ cup UNBLEACHED WHITE
FLOUR
¾ cup double-strength chicken
broth, homemade or canned

¼ cup light cream (or evaporated
milk)
2 tablespoons Chablis, or other
dry white wine
¼ teaspoon SEA SALT
⅛ teaspoon ground white pepper

GARNISH:

1 tablespoon snipped fresh parsley

¼ cup grated Parmesan cheese
Paprika

Cook broccoli conventionally, or slash package of frozen spears and microwave on a paper towel for 7 minutes
on full power. Let stand.

Bone chicken, skin and cut in 1-inch pieces. (Neatness
doesn't count for this as ragged edges will never be noticed
and the trimmings will be reserved for making chicken
broth.) Place in 1½-quart flame-proof casserole. Marinate
in mixture of arrowroot, sesame oil and Marsala. Let
stand at least 15 minutes.

While chicken is marinating, make cream sauce: heat oil
and margarine in a small saucepan over low heat. Stir in
flour, broth and cream. Cook and stir until thickened and
bubbling—6 to 7 minutes. Whisk in white wine, salt and
pepper.

TO MICROWAVE CREAM SAUCE: Place oil and
margarine in 4-cup glass measure and stir in flour.
Microwave 1 minute on full power. Stir in broth and
cream. Microwave 3 minutes on full power, stirring
once. Whisk in white wine, salt and pepper.

Stir chicken in marinade, cover and cook over low heat until boiling. Remove cover and cook and stir about 5 minutes, or until chicken pieces are firm and white.

TO MICROWAVE CHICKEN & MARINADE: Microwave, covered, for 2 minutes on full power. Stir and microwave 1 minute without cover.

Stir chicken and drippings into sauce with parsley. Arrange broccoli spears in casserole in which chicken was cooked. Pour sauce mixture over broccoli. Sprinkle with Parmesan cheese and a drift of paprika. Reheat before serving, if necessary.

SUPER-NUTRITION VARIATION:

• Stir in 1 teaspoon DOLOMITE POWDER with the broth
• Combine the Parmesan cheese with: ½ teaspoon B-COMPLEX POWDER
⅛ teaspoon C-TRATE contents of 1 10,000 IU SUPER DRY A & D capsule

Yield: 4 servings

CHICKEN & NOODLES, ITALIAN-STYLE

In Italy, pasta is served with a wide variety of sauces, only a few of which contain tomatoes. Use whole wheat spaghetti instead of noodles if you'd rather, for this meal-in-a-dish that has a real Italian flavor plus an amazing amount of vitamins and minerals—and requires very few preparation minutes.

1 large chicken breast (1 pound)	¼ large green bell pepper, chopped
2 tablespoons dry white wine or apple juice	¼ pound fresh mushrooms, cleaned and sliced
4 ounces dry whole wheat noodles	4 tablespoons UNBLEACHED WHITE FLOUR
1 tablespoon COLD PRESSED VIRGIN OLIVE OIL	2 tablespoons SOY FLOUR
1 tablespoon safflower margarine	½ teaspoon crushed, dried Italian seasoning
½ medium onion, chopped	

½ teaspoon SEA SALT
½ teaspoon paprika
⅛ teaspoon ground black pepper
⅛ teaspoon garlic powder
1½ cups water

½ cup non-instant SKIM MILK POWDER
¼ cup grated Parmesan cheese
1 tablespoon snipped fresh parsley

Skin and bone chicken. Reserve trimmings for making broth and cut meat into ¾-inch pieces. Combine with wine in a small bowl, cover and let stand.

Cook noodles in boiling, salted water; drain (rinse, if desired), cover and let stand.

Sauté onion and bell pepper in the oil and margarine for 3 or 4 minutes. Stir in mushrooms and sauté about 5 minutes—until vegetables are limp but not browned. Stir in white flour, soy flour, Italian seasoning, salt, paprika, black pepper and garlic powder. Blend water with skim milk powder and stir in. Cook and stir until mixture is beginning to simmer and is slightly thickened. Stir in chicken pieces with liquid and cook until chicken is firm and white. Add noodles, grated cheese and parsley. Stir to combine and heat to serving temperature.

TO MICROWAVE: Skin and bone chicken and cut into ¾-inch pieces. Combine with wine in a small bowl, cover and let stand.

Combine noodles with 4 cups boiling, salted water in a 2-quart casserole. Add 1 teaspoon oil, cover and microwave on full power for 3 minutes—or until boiling. Stir, leave uncovered and microwave for 3 minutes on full power. Stir, cover and let stand for 5 minutes before draining.

In the 2-quart casserole, combine onion, bell pepper, oil and margarine. Cover and microwave for 2 minutes on full power. Stir in mushrooms and microwave, uncovered, for 3 minutes. Stir in flours and seasonings. Blend water with skim milk powder and stir in. Microwave, uncovered, for 5 minutes on full power—stirring once each minute. Stir in chicken and wine and microwave 5 minutes on full power, stirring once. (Chicken should be firm and sauce thickened and almost boiling.) Stir in noodles, grated cheese and parsley. Microwave just to serving temperature.

SUPER-NUTRITION VARIATION:

Combine with the Parmesan cheese before adding to the casserole:
- 1 tablespoon LECITHIN GRANULES
- Contents of 1 DAILY B-COMPLEX capsule
- Contents of 1 10,000 IU SUPER DRY A & D capsule
- ⅛ teaspoon C-TRATE

Yield: 6 servings

CITY CHICKEN DINNER

Country cooks may have time for "stringing" green beans and slow-roasting or long simmering their whole chickens, but city cooks can achieve the same results with chicken breasts and frozen vegetables . . . and include some supplemental vitamins as well.

2 whole chicken breasts (1¾ pounds) split and skinned
1¼ teaspoons SPIKE
1 teaspoon paprika
1 teaspoon crushed, dried parsley
¼ teaspoon crushed, dried tarragon
1 pound potatoes (4 medium) peeled and cut in 2-inch pieces

1 10-ounce package frozen, cut green beans, defrosted enough to separate
1 medium onion, quartered and sliced
½ cup sliced fresh mushrooms or one 2 ¾-ounce can mushrooms, drained

Wash chicken and pat dry. In a small dish, combine Spike, paprika, parsley and tarragon and sprinkle on both sides of the chicken. Place chicken pieces meaty-side down in a 2-quart casserole. Add potatoes, green beans, onion and mushrooms. Cover and bake in a preheated 375 degree oven for 45 minutes. Turn chicken pieces, replace cover and continue baking until all are tender—about 15 minutes.

TO MICROWAVE: Wash chicken and pat dry. In a small dish, combine Spike, paprika, parsley and tarragon and sprinkle on both sides of the chicken. Place chicken pieces in the corners of a $10 \times 10 \times 2$-inch casserole and arrange potatoes, green beans, onion and mushrooms around and over the chicken. Cover with a lid or plastic wrap and microwave on full power for 15 minutes. Stir and turn chicken pieces. Cover and microwave on full power for 10 minutes, turning dish after 5 minutes. Let stand for 5 minutes before serving.

WITH 3-4 QUART PRESSURE COOKER: Arrange potatoes in the bottom of the pressure cooker and pour in 1 cup of water. Wash chicken and pat dry. Combine Spike, paprika, parsley and tarragon and sprinkle on both sides of the chicken. Place chicken breasts over the potatoes, then add remaining ingredients. Close cover of the cooker and put pressure control in place. When pressure is reached and control jiggles, cook for 15 minutes. Reduce pressure immediately.

If desired, the cooking liquid from the pressure cooker can be thickened to serve as a gravy for the potatoes: blend 2 tablespoons ARROWROOT with 1 tablespoon of water and stir into the liquid. Cook in the open cooker until boiling and thickened.

SUPER-NUTRITION VARIATION:

Combine with the Spike, paprika, parsley and tarragon:
- ⅛ teaspoon C-TRATE
- contents of one 5,000 IU SUPER DRY A & D capsule
- contents of one DAILY B-COMPLEX capsule

Yield: 4 servings

MEDITERRANEAN CHICKEN DINNER

For an extraordinarily delicious Eastern Mediterranean dinner, serve with Stir-fried Cucumbers & Onions and warm Pocket Bread (recipes on pages 143 & 181) adding stuffed eggplant or zucchini to the menu, if desired. When you have cooked garbanzos on hand, you can microwave this same exotic dish in twenty minutes—including the five minutes of preliminary preparation time.

1 cup dry GARBANZOS
1 quart water
½ teaspoon INSTANT LIQUID TENDERIZER
1 pound chicken breasts (1 large whole breast or 3 small halves)
1 tablespoon COLD PRESSED SESAME OIL
1 medium onion, chopped
1 medium carrot, scraped or peeled and grated
½ cup BULGUR WHEAT
1½ teaspoons SEA SALT
1 teaspoon paprika
½ teaspoon ground coriander
¼ teaspoon garlic powder

⅛ teaspoon ground red pepper (cayenne)
2 tablespoons RAW WHEAT GERM
2 tablespoons non-instant SKIM MILK POWDER
¼ teaspoon C-TRATE
½ cup Soymilk (recipe on page 135) or 2 tablespoons soy flour plus water to make ½ cup
2 tablespoons snipped fresh parsley
2 tablespoons diced, canned pimiento
Garnish: 12 cherry tomatoes plus additional snipped parsley

Wash garbanzos under running water. Combine in a heavy kettle with water and tenderizer. Let stand 5 minutes. Bring to a full boil for 2 minutes, cover and let stand for 1 hour.

Skin chicken and place in the kettle with the garbanzos. Bring to boiling, reduce heat and simmer, covered, until chicken is tender—about 30 minutes. Remove chicken, cover garbanzos and continue simmering for 45 minutes.

Meanwhile, discard chicken bones, cut meat in half-inch dice and refrigerate.

Heat sesame oil in a skillet and stir in onion, carrot and bulgur. Cook and stir until onion is limp, then stir into garbanzos with salt, paprika, coriander, garlic and red pepper. Cover and simmer for 20 minutes, or until garbanzos are tender.

Combine wheat germ, skim milk powder and C-Trate. Blend in soymilk and stir into garbanzo mixture. Cook and stir until boiling, then add chicken, parsley and pimiento. Let stand 5 minutes over the heat, then transfer to serving bowl. Garnish with a ring of halved cherry tomatoes and a sprinkling of snipped parsley.

TO MICROWAVE WITH PRE-COOKED GAR-BANZOS:

1 medium onion
1 medium carrot, scraped or peeled
1 tablespoon COLD PRESSED SESAME OIL
½ cup BULGUR WHEAT
1 teaspoon SEA SALT
1 teaspoon paprika
½ teaspoon ground coriander
¼ teaspoon garlic powder
⅛ teaspoon ground red pepper (cayenne)
1 cup chicken broth, home-made or canned
1 pound chicken breasts
2 tablespoons RAW WHEAT GERM

2 tablespoons non-instant SKIM MILK POWDER
2 tablespoons SOY FLOUR
¼ teaspoon C-TRATE
2 cups cooked, drained GARBANZOS, plus ½ cup of their cooking liquid
2 tablespoons snipped fresh parsley
2 tablespoons diced, canned pimiento
Garnish: 12 cherry tomatoes plus additional snipped parsley

Mince onion and carrot with food processor or chop and shred by hand. Combine with the oil in a 2-quart casserole. Cover and microwave on full power for 3 minutes.

Stir in bulgur with salt, paprika, coriander, garlic, red pepper and chicken broth. Cover and microwave on full power for 8 minutes.

Bone and skin chicken breasts. Cut into ¾-inch pieces and stir into the boiling mixture. Cover and microwave for 2 minutes on full power.

Combine wheat germ, skim milk powder, soy flour, C-Trate and the half-cup of garbanzo cooking liquid. Stir in with garbanzos. Cover and microwave on full power for 2 minutes. Stir in parsley and pimiento.

Serve in the cooking casserole, garnish with a ring of halved cherry tomatoes and a sprinkling of snipped parsley.

SUBSTITUTIONS:
● Omit coriander, garlic powder and ground red pepper. Add 1 tablespoon curry powder with the bulgur and vegetables
● Omit soymilk or soyflour and water. Blend ¼ cup water with ¼ cup YOGURT and stir into the wheat-germ mixture before adding to garbanzos

VARIATION: *VEGETARIAN MEDITERRANEAN DINNER*
● Omit chicken and prepare as directed, allowing the garbanzos to simmer for 1 hour and 15 minutes before adding the bulgur and vegetables if preparing on the stove top.
● Stir in ¼ cup SUNFLOWER-SESAME BUTTER with the parsley and pimiento

Yield: 6 servings

MAIN DISH MILLET PILAF

Millet is a delightfully versatile grain that, happily, is becoming better known in the United States. Millet isn't a newcomer by any means; it was one of the first cereal grasses to be domesticated by man and has been a food staple for much of the world's population for thousands of years. Ancient Romans made their bread from ground millet and wheat, and it still is used as a flour for cakes and puddings in Africa, Egypt and India. It is higher in protein, lower in carbohydrates, and contains more of all eight of the essential amino acids, more fiber, iron, potassium, magnesium, thiamine and riboflavin than either white or brown rice. With its light and fluffy texture, millet makes a flavorful change from rice in this pilaf, and may be used as a rice-substitute in most dishes.

1 medium onion, chopped	1¾ cups boiling chicken broth,
1 tablespoon safflower margarine	homemade or canned
½ cup HULLED MILLET	¼ pound fresh mushrooms*
½ teaspoon SEA SALT	1 cup cooked, diced chicken
½ teaspoon KELP SEASONING	

Melt margarine in saucepan over medium heat and cook onion until limp but not brown, stirring frequently. Stir in millet, salt and kelp. Add broth, cover and simmer over low heat for 45 minutes. Stir several times during the last half of the cooking time to prevent sticking. Wash mushrooms and roll in paper towel to dry. Slice in processor, or on thick-slicer of hand grater. Stir in and cook 10 minutes. Stir in chicken, cover and heat just to serving temperature over low heat.

TO MICROWAVE: Combine margarine with onion in 1½-quart casserole and microwave on full power for 2 minutes, uncovered. Stir in millet, salt and kelp. Add broth. Cover and microwave on full power for 25 minutes, stirring after 15 minutes. Wash mushrooms and roll in paper towel to dry. Slice in processor or on thick-slicer of hand grater. Stir in, cover and microwave on full power for 5 minutes. Stir in chicken, cover and microwave just to serving temperature.

Yield: 4 servings

---

*One 4-ounce can drained mushrooms may be substituted and the liquid included as part of the broth.

DELICATESSEN CHICKEN WITH BROTH

A beautifully simple way to make a succulently tender "rotisseried bird" out of a whole fryer, and gain at least a quart of exceptionally rich chicken broth with more nutritional value than the canned variety.

1 whole, 3-pound frying chicken
1 pound (approximately) reserved chicken wings, necks, bones and skin
2 celery tops with leaves
½ small onion stuck with one whole clove
3 or 4 sprigs fresh parsley or 1 teaspoon dried parsley
1 large carrot, thinly sliced or chopped
1 teaspoon APPLE CIDER VINEGAR
1½ teaspoons SEA SALT
1 teaspoon VEGETABLE SALAD POWDER
1 teaspoon GRANULATED KELP
½ teaspoon whole peppercorns
¼ teaspoon poultry seasoning
1 recipe Rotisserie Magic (recipe on page 155)

Rinse the chicken and place the celery tops, onion and parsley sprigs in the cavity. Tie the drumsticks together with string. Place a layer of the chicken bones in the bottom of a 4 or 5-quart Dutch oven or kettle. Add the whole chicken and arrange the remaining chicken pieces around it to hold the wings close to the body. Add the rest of the ingredients (including dried parsley, if used) and fill the kettle with warm water to cover the chicken or to come within 1½ inches of the top. Cover and bring to boiling. Reduce heat and simmer, covered, until chicken is tender—2½ to 3 hours. If chicken is not completely submerged in the cooking liquid, turn it over after 1½ hours of simmering.

WITH MICROWAVE OVEN: Prepare as directed, using a 4 or 5-quart casserole. Cover and microwave on full power for 45 minutes, turning chicken over after 25 minutes. Let stand for 10 minutes and test chicken—a very cold or slightly larger bird may require an additional 15 minutes of microwaving.

WITH SLOW-COOKER: The slow-cooker will simmer the chicken all day and have it ready for a quick brushing with Rotisserie Magic before presentation as a hot entree for dinner. For a delicious cold bird, reverse the timing and refrigerate the chicken before you leave in the morning. Prepare as directed, using a 3½ to 4-quart slow-cooker. Cover, set on Low and cook for 6 to 9 hours. The timing can be regulated by the temperature of the chicken pieces and the water—if the cooker will be unattended for longer than 8 hours, have the chicken frosty cold and include a handful of ice cubes with cold water to cover.

When the chicken is tender, lift it to a cutting board and remove the vegetables from the cavity. Discard them as well as the carrot—they will have given their all to the broth. If desired, remove the skin from all but the wings of the chicken. (The fat will have cooked away, so this is an esthetic choice.)

Prepare Rotisserie Magic and brush over all surfaces of the chicken with a pastry brush. For immediate serving, insert a meat thermometer in a thigh and heat to 140 degrees in a preheated 375 degree oven, or use a microwave temperature probe or thermometer and microwave on full power. If the chicken is to be served cold, bake for 10 minutes or microwave for 3 minutes. Before refrigerating the chicken, crumple a paper towel and insert it in the cavity to absorb any moisture—then be sure to remove it before serving!

Yield: 4 servings

CHICKEN BROTH:

Empty the contents of the cooking container into a large sieve or colander over a mixing bowl. Shred off any usable meat, then discard bones, skin and vegetables. Pour the broth through a fine-mesh sieve into a refrigerator container. Chill until the fat forms an easily removed layer on top of the broth. Spoon the clear, jellied broth into small containers for freezing if you are not going to use it within a day or two. The cloudy layer at the bottom may be included in meat loaves or casserole dishes in order to avoid wasting any of the nutrients.

Yield: Approximately 4 cups

AVOCADO-TUNA AMANDINE

A nutrition-packed combination dish for family or guests; a salad and fruit dessert completes the meal, even when the vegetarian version is served. The bit of dolomite maintains the proper proportions for the calcium-magnesium and phosphorus while the vitamin C acts as an antioxidant in case any harmful chemicals are lurking in the canned tuna.

1½ cups water*
½ teaspoon SEA SALT
1 teaspoon COLD PRESSED ALMOND OIL

½ cup raw LONG-GRAIN BROWN RICE

CREAM SAUCE

3 tablespoons COLD PRESSED SAFFLOWER OIL
¼ cup UNBLEACHED WHITE FLOUR
¼ teaspoon DOLOMITE POWDER
1¼ cups chicken broth, homemade or canned
⅓ cup non-instant SKIM MILK POWDER

½ teaspoon VEGETABLE SALAD POWDER
¼ teaspoon natural celery salt
1 7-ounce can tuna, drained
1 large avocado (8 ounces)
1 teaspoon fresh lemon juice
¼ teaspoon C-TRATE
2 green onions, medium size, with crisp green tops
2 tablespoons slivered almonds

Bring water, salt and almond oil to a boil in medium saucepan. Stir in rice, cover and cook 40 minutes over low heat. Stir and let stand, covered.

> **TO MICROWAVE:** Combine water, salt and almond oil in 1½-quart casserole. Cover and microwave 25 minutes on full power, stirring after 15 minutes. Let stand, covered.

While rice is standing, make sauce: Heat safflower oil in saucepan, stir in flour and cook 1 minute. Stir in dolomite, broth, dry milk, Vegetable Salad Powder and celery salt. Cook and stir over low heat until thickened and bubbling.

---

*For more tender rice: Add ¼ cup water and cook until as tender as desired.

TO MICROWAVE SAUCE: Combine safflower oil and flour in a 4-cup glass measure and microwave 1 minute on full power. Stir in dolomite, broth, dry milk, Vegetable Salad Powder and celery salt. Microwave 5 minutes on full power, stirring after 2 minutes, then once each minute.

Drain tuna, break into pieces and stir into sauce. Peel and core avocado. Cut in ½-inch cubes and toss with lemon juice and C-Trate. Stir into sauce.

Thinly slice green onions and stir into rice. Cover and cook over low heat for 5 minutes (or microwave for 3 minutes). Stir sauce mixture into rice. Sprinkle almonds over casserole and heat until bubbling: 20 minutes in a preheated, 375 degree conventional oven, or 5 minutes in a microwave oven on full power.

VARIATIONS: *VEGETARIAN AVOCADO AMANDINE*

- Cook rice as directed
- Make the Cream Sauce with vegetable stock instead of chicken broth (If no broth is on hand, stir additional Vegetable Salad Powder into hot water.)
- Omit tuna
- Stir in with avocado: 2 hard-cooked eggs, chopped
  3 ounces shredded natural cheddar cheese
- Increase slivered almonds to ¼ cup
- Sprinkle 2 tablespoons Imitation Bacon Bits over the top of the casserole.
- Heat until bubbling, as for Avocado-Tuna Amandine.

Yield: 4 servings

FILLET OF SOLE DELLA ROBBIA

A healthful, spectacular dish for a special luncheon or an impressive buffet—and superlatively easy to prepare, especially since it may be completed well in advance of serving time.

⅓ cup chicken broth, homemade or canned

⅓ cup dry white wine or apple juice

⅛ teaspoon C-TRATE

4 sole fillets (1 pound)

⅛ teaspoon SEA SALT

1¼ teaspoons PURE GELATIN

Curly leaf lettuce or endive

1 cup cantaloupe balls

½ cup seedless green grapes

½ cup fresh or frozen, unsweetened blueberries

½ fresh lime, cut in 4 lengthwise wedges

Bleu Cheese-Sour Cream Dressing (recipe on page 29)

Pour broth and wine in a skillet, heat to boiling and stir in C-Trate. Roll fillets from the wide end and wrap in cheesecloth, tying ends with string to hold in place. Place in hot liquid, cover and simmer for 10 minutes, until fish are solid, turning rolls over after 5 minutes.

TO MICROWAVE: Combine broth with wine in a shallow, 1-quart casserole. Cover and microwave for 2 minutes on full power. Stir in C-Trate. Roll fish fillets from the wide end and wrap each one in cheesecloth, tying ends with string to hold in place. Place the fish in the boiling liquid, cover and microwave for 3 minutes, turning dish after 2 minutes.

Lift fish from the liquid and cool. Strain cooking liquid and let cool. Combine gelatin with salt and stir in half the liquid (⅓ cup). Heat to simmering and stir to dissolve gelatin. Stir in remaining liquid and chill until slightly thickened, but still liquid—about 15 minutes.

Remove cheesecloth from fish and spoon on the gelatin mixture, completely covering the fish rolls. Chill until the gelatin is set, then spoon on a second layer, warming the aspic a little if necessary. Chill fish for several hours before serving.

To Serve: Place fish in the center of a large, round plate and surround with a wreath of lettuce. Decorate with cantaloupe, grapes, blueberries and lime wedges. Spoon a little Bleu Cheese Dressing over the fish and pass the remainder in a separate bowl.

To Prepare Ahead: Refrigerate aspic-covered fish rolls in a 2-inch deep covered container for up to 24 hours. The cantaloupe balls may be frozen with a sprinkling of C-Trate, and the grapes and blueberries frozen on cookie sheets for loose-pack freezer storage. Arrange the fruits on the lettuce while still frozen, cover the entire platter with plastic wrap and refrigerate for an hour or so before serving.

Yield: 4 servings

CREOLE JAMBALAYA

First cousin to a paella and twice-removed from "Hoppin' John," this Jambalaya is ideal for anticipated guests or busy days as it may be prepared in installments or completed and refrigerated for a day before heating and serving.

1 tablespoon COLD PRESSED ALL BLEND OIL

2 medium onions, divided

½ teaspoon chili powder

⅛ teaspoon garlic powder

⅔ cup raw BROWN RICE

1⅓ cups chicken broth, homemade or canned*

1 large green bell pepper cut in ½-inch squares

2 medium ribs celery, thinly sliced

1 tablespoon safflower margarine

1 cup Slow & Easy Tomato Sauce (recipe on page 160)

6 ounces shelled, cleaned shrimp, cut in half if large

½ teaspoon SEA SALT

⅛ teaspoon freshly ground black pepper

1½ cups cooked, drained dried BLACK-EYED PEAS (cooking directions on page 124)

1½ cups diced, cooked chicken

2 tablespoons diced, canned pimiento

2 tablespoons snipped fresh parsley

Chop 1 onion and sauté with oil, chili powder and garlic powder until onion is limp. Stir in rice, then add

---

*For tender, fluffy rice, increase the broth to 1½ cups and cook until all the liquid is absorbed—about 20 minutes on the stove, 6 to 8 minutes in the microwave.

broth. Cover and bring to boiling. Stir, reduce heat, cover and simmer 45 minutes. Let stand, covered.

Chop remaining onion and sauté in a small skillet with the green pepper and celery until vegetables are limp but not browned. Stir into rice with Tomato sauce, shrimp, salt and pepper. Cover and simmer about 10 minutes—until shrimp are cooked. Stir in black-eyed peas, chicken, pimiento and parsley. Cover and heat to serving temperature.

> **TO MICROWAVE:** Chop 1 onion and combine with oil, chili and garlic powder in a 2-quart casserole. Cover and microwave on full power for 2 minutes. Stir in rice, then add broth. Cover and microwave on full power until boiling—about 5 minutes. Stir, replace cover and microwave on Defrost (half power) for 20 minutes. Let stand, covered.
>
> Chop remaining onion and combine in a 4-cup glass measure with green pepper, celery and margarine. Microwave on full power for 3 minutes, stirring once. Stir into the rice with Tomato sauce, shrimp, salt and pepper. Cover and microwave 5 minutes—until shrimp are cooked. Stir in black-eyed peas, chicken, pimiento and parsley. Cover and microwave on full power until serving temperature.

Serve garnished with lemon wedges, pimiento strips and parsley sprigs.

Yield: 6 servings

VEGETARIAN VARIATION: *BLACK-EYED JAMBALAYA*

Delicious even without any meat, chicken or shrimp, the amino acids in the rice and black-eyed peas complement each other to form complete proteins. (The peas provide the extra isoleucine *and lysine needed by the rice which furnishes tryptophan for the peas.**)

Prepare as directed, except:
- Substitute vegetable broth or salted water for the chicken broth
- Substitute Quick & Easy Tomato Sauce made with water (recipe on page 158), for the Slow & Easy Tomato Sauce.
- Omit shrimp and chicken.

Each of the six servings contains 9½ grams of protein which can be augmented by sprinkling grated Parmesan or shredded cheddar cheese atop the hot casserole.

SUPER-NUTRITION VARIATION FOR EITHER VERSION:

- Add with the salt and pepper: ½ teaspoon paprika
      ¼ teaspoon C-TRATE
      contents of 1 DAILY B-
      COMPLEX Capsule

---

*David Reuben, Everything You Always Wanted To Know About Nutrition, Simon and Schuster, 1978.

NUT-CRUSTED TROUT

Oven frying makes these fat-reduced, splatter-free, crusty-brown trout an easily prepared super-spectacular for special meals. To reinforce your title as "resident gourmet," serve with a salad, steamed asparagus spears and freshly warmed rolls. For heartier appetites you could add parsleyed potatoes and a dessert.

4 whole rainbow trout,* dressed (1½ pounds)

2 tablespoons Seasoned Flour (recipe on page 154)

1 large egg

2 tablespoons milk

⅔ cup walnuts, ground

⅓ cup RAW WHEAT GERM

¼ teaspoon paprika

2 tablespoons safflower margarine

2 tablespoons COLD PRESSED ALL BLEND OIL

Wipe fish with a dampened paper towel and dredge with

Seasoned Flour. Beat egg with milk and dip each fish to coat all over.

Grind nuts with wheat germ and paprika in a processor or blender and roll fish in the mixture.

Place margarine and oil in a baking pan just large enough to hold the trout in a single layer. Heat in the oven until bubbling and swirl to blend. Lay fish in the pan and turn to coat. Bake in a preheated 425 degree oven for 10 minutes, uncovered. Turn fish with a spatula and bake until fish flakes easily—5 to 10 minutes.

> **TO MICROWAVE:** Coat fish with Seasoned Flour, egg and milk mixture. Roll in the walnuts which have been ground with the wheat germ and paprika. Place margarine and oil in a baking dish just large enough to hold the trout in a single layer. Microwave for 45 seconds on full power and swirl to blend. Lay trout in the warm dish and turn to coat. Microwave, uncovered, for 5 minutes on full power, turning dish after 3 minutes. If fish does not flake easily, microwave for an additional minute.

Serve garnished with fresh parsley and lemon wedges.

Yield: 4 servings

---

*If fish are frozen, defrost in the refrigerator, in a bowl of cold water, or speed the process by microwaving on half power for 2 minutes and then completing the defrosting in a bowl of cold water.

SALMON NEWBURG WITH PEAS

Another old favorite with a nutritional update. Serve over Oatmeal Waffles (recipe on page 177) and accompany with steamed broccoli and sliced tomatoes for a quick-fix luncheon or supper with visual as well as taste appeal. (Meal totals are included in the Nutritional Analysis Tables.)

1 tablespoon COLD PRESSED ALL BLEND OIL
1 tablespoon safflower margarine
3 tablespoons non-instant SKIM MILK POWDER
2 tablespoons WHOLE WHEAT PASTRY FLOUR
1 tablespoon SOY FLOUR
½ teaspoon SPIKE
¼ teaspoon paprika
⅔ cup water
1 cup frozen peas, defrosted enough to separate
1 egg yolk
⅓ cup light cream (half-and-half) or evaporated milk
8 ounces canned sockeye salmon with liquid (one-half of 1-pound can)
2 tablespoons LECITHIN GRANULES
1 tablespoon cream sherry or apple juice
2 tablespoons chopped, canned pimiento
⅛ teaspoon C-TRATE

Melt margarine with oil in a 2-quart saucepan over low heat. Blend skim milk powder, pastry flour, soy flour, Spike and paprika in a small bowl and gradually whisk in water. Stir into the warm oil and margarine. Cook and stir until thickened. Stir in peas and cook until boiling.

Blend egg yolk with cream and stir into the hot mixture. Heat to simmering. Stir in salmon with liquid, lecithin granules, wine, chopped pimiento and C-Trate. Heat just to serving temperature.

TO MICROWAVE: Place oil and margarine in a 4-cup glass measure and microwave on full power for 30 seconds. Blend skim milk powder, pastry flour, soy flour, Spike and paprika in a small bowl and gradually whisk in water. Stir into the warm oil and margarine. Microwave for 2 minutes on full power, stirring once. Stir in peas and microwave for 2 minutes.

Blend egg yolk with cream and stir into the hot mixture. Microwave on full power for 2 minutes. Stir in remaining ingredients and heat just to serving temperature.

Serve over toast points or assemble "waffle shortcakes" by placing half a waffle on each plate, spooning on salmon mixture, covering with the other half of the waffle and topping with salmon.   **Yield: 4 servings**

MACARONI & CHEESE

*Even this mundane dish can be flavorful enough for gourmet
entertaining, and nutritious enough for the health-conscious.
Using whole-grain macaroni adds iron and B vitamins; the carrot adds color, potassium and vitamin A; while the liquid lecithin, combined with that in the soy flour and egg, takes care of
the fats; and the green chiles provide pizzaz.*

Macaroni:

8 ounces (1¾ cups) uncooked
  whole wheat macaroni
  boiling water

1 teaspoon *each* SEA SALT and
  COLD PRESSED ALL BLEND
  OIL

Cheese Sauce:

2 tablespoons COLD PRESSED
  ALL BLEND OIL
1 tablespoon safflower margarine
¼ cup UNBLEACHED WHITE
  FLOUR
2 tablespoons SOY FLOUR
1 teaspoon SEA SALT
1½ cups water, divided
12 ounces natural, sharp cheddar
  cheese, cut in half-inch cubes
  (2¼ cups)

1 large carrot
1 large egg
3 tablespoons non-instant SKIM
  MILK POWDER
1 tablespoon LIQUID LECI-
  THIN
½ of 4-ounce can chopped green
  chiles

Cook macaroni in 2 quarts of boiling water with the
teaspoon of salt and oil. Drain in a colander and rinse, if
desired, to remove excess starch. (If you are counting
carbohydrates, cook the macaroni for an extra minute or so
before draining and rinsing to reduce the starch by one-
fourth.) Let stand, covered.

Melt margarine with oil in a saucepan and stir in the
white flour, soy flour and salt. Stir in water and cook over
low heat until thickened and bubbling, stirring constantly.
Stir in cheese, cover and let stand for the cheese to melt.

Scrape or peel the carrot and cut into 1-inch chunks.
Liquefy in an electric blender with the remaining half-cup
of water. (Or shred as finely as possible by hand.) Add
egg, skim milk powder and lecithin and blend until smooth.

111

Stir into the cheese sauce with the chiles, then stir in drained macaroni.

Transfer to a 2-quart casserole and bake in a preheated 375 degree oven for 30 minutes.

TO MICROWAVE: Stir macaroni into 1 quart of boiling water in a 2-quart casserole with the teaspoon of salt and oil. Cover and microwave on full power for 3 minutes, or until fully boiling. Stir, cover, set control on Defrost (half power) and microwave for 10 minutes. Let stand 2 minutes.

Drain in a colander and rinse, if desired, to remove excess starch. (If you are counting carbohydrates, cook the macaroni for an extra minute or so before draining and rinsing to reduce the starch by one-fourth.) Let stand, covered.

Place oil and margarine in the casserole in which the macaroni was cooked. Microwave for 30 seconds on full power, then stir in white flour, soy flour and salt. Stir in 1 cup of the water and microwave on full power for about 4 minutes, stirring once each minute. (Sauce should be thickened and bubbling.) Add cheese, cover and microwave for 1 minute. Let stand for a minute or so to melt cheese.

Scrape or peel the carrot and cut into 1-inch chunks. Liquefy in an electric blender with the remaining half-cup of water. (Or shred as finely as possible on a hand grater.) Add egg, skim milk powder and lecithin and blend until smooth. Stir into the cheese sauce with the chiles, then stir in drained macaroni.

Microwave, uncovered, for 10 minutes on full power, rotating dish once. For a crusty topping, brown the microwaved dish for 2 or 3 minutes under a conventional broiler or microwave browning unit.

SUPER-NUTRITION VARIATION:

- Add to blender with carrot: ¼ teaspoon B-COMPLEX
POWDER

⅛ teaspoon C-TRATE

- Combine and sprinkle atop the casserole before the final baking or microwaving: 2 tablespoons grated Parmesan cheese
2 tablespoons RICE BRAN
¼ teaspoon paprika

NOTE: For two 4-serving casseroles, place half the prepared Macaroni & Cheese in a metal pan and freeze before the final baking or microwaving. For convenience, freeze half the super-nutrition topping in a plastic bag and overwrap with the macaroni. Sprinkle on the defrosted casserole just before the final heating. **Yield: Eight ¾-cup servings**

IMPERIAL POTTAGE

A dish very similar to this, but more complex,* was served Julius Caesar in imperial Rome. The cooks of that era had just been accorded professional status and vied with each other in developing a highly sophisticated cuisine utilizing regional vegetables and herbs along with the expensively imported foods and spices. Unfortunately, they cooked their vegetables in copper pots and then added soda to intensify the colors—a combination which would have destroyed all vitamin C and thus may have contributed to the decline of that great empire!

1 tablespoon COLD PRESSED ALL BLEND OIL
1 medium onion, chopped
¼ cup BARLEY
2 cups water
⅓ cup dry split peas, rinsed
⅓ cup dry LENTILS, rinsed
½ teaspoon SEA SALT
2 cups chopped raw cabbage
⅓ cup chopped green onion tops
¼ teaspoon crushed, dried oregano
⅛ teaspoon crushed fennel seed

⅛ teaspoon garlic powder
2 tablespoons dry white wine or water
1 teaspoon COLD PRESSED OLIVE OIL
1¼ cups drained, cooked GARBANZOS (cooking directions are on page 124)
2 tablespoons snipped fresh parsley
⅛ teaspoon freshly ground black pepper

---

*The original version included chopped beets and dill; used leeks instead of onions; coriander in place of parsley; and added generous amounts of oil and wine along with some herbs no longer available. (*Cookery and Dining in Imperial Rome*, Apicius [80 B.C. to A.D. 40] Vehling translation, Dover Publications, New York, 1977).

In a medium saucepan, sauté onion in the tablespoon of oil until limp but not browned. Stir in barley and water and bring to a full boil. Slowly add peas and lentils without stopping the boiling. Reduce heat, cover and simmer for 30 minutes. Stir in salt, cover and continue simmering until all are done—about 15 minutes—and liquid is absorbed.

In a small saucepan, combine cabbage, green onion tops, oregano, fennel, garlic powder, wine and olive oil. Cover tightly and cook until cabbage is tender-crisp, stirring when necessary to prevent browning.

Stir cabbage mixture into the cooked legumes and add garbanzos, parsley and black pepper. Heat to serving temperature.

TO MICROWAVE: Add ½ teaspoon INSTANT LIQUID TENDERIZER to the 2 cups of water and pour over the rinsed lentils and split peas. Let stand for 15 minutes.

In a 2-quart casserole, combine chopped onion with the tablespoon of oil. Cover and microwave on full power for 3 minutes. Stir in barley, then add the soaked lentils and peas with their liquid. Cover and microwave on full power for 15 minutes, stirring after 10 minutes. Stir in salt, cover and microwave for 5 minutes. Test and microwave an additional 5 minutes if the vegetables are not tender and/or all the liquid has not been absorbed.

In a 4-cup glass measure, combine cabbage, onion tops, oregano, fennel, garlic and water or wine. Cover and microwave on full power until cabbage is tender-crisp—approximately 5 minutes—stirring after 3 minutes.

Stir cabbage mixture into the cooked legumes with the garbanzos, parsley and black pepper. Microwave, if necessary, to heat to serving temperature.

SUPER-NUTRITION VARIATION:

- Add ½ teaspoon KELP SEASONING with the salt
- Add with the pepper: ⅛ teaspoon C-TRATE
  contents of one DAILY B-COM-
  PLEX capsule
  contents of one 5,000 IU SUPER
  DRY A & D capsule

Yield: 4 generous servings

ONION QUICHE

More character (and vitamins) than the usual entree custard with bacon bits, this onion quiche is an inexpensive spectacular for company meals or family fare. The super-nutrition variation makes a completely balanced snack, or can serve as a mini-meal with the addition of a salad. The refrigerated wedges may be warmed in a microwave or toaster oven, if desired, but are equally delicious when served cold.

½ recipe for Wheat Pastry, page 223
1 pound onions, chopped (4 cups)
1 tablespoon safflower margarine
1 tablespoon COLD-PRESSED ALL BLEND OIL
½ cup sour cream
3 tablespoons non-instant SKIM MILK POWDER
1 tablespoon UNBLEACHED WHITE FLOUR
¾ teaspoon SEA SALT
⅛ teaspoon ground white pepper
½ cup (2 ounces) shredded Swiss cheese
½ cup water
2 large eggs
Garnish: 2 tablespoons shredded Swiss cheese
⅛ teaspoon nutmeg

Roll pastry between 12-inch squares of waxed paper and line a 9-inch pie pan. Flute rim and set aside.

Chop onions by hand or in food processor. Sauté with margarine and oil until onions are golden. Set aside.

In food processor or mixing bowl, combine sour cream with skim milk powder, flour, salt and pepper. Chop cheese in half-inch chunks and add to the processor, or shred and add to mixing bowl. Process or stir until blended. Add water and eggs and process or beat. Stir into the cooked onions.

Pour into the unbaked pastry shell and sprinkle with the 2 tablespoons of cheese and the nutmeg. Bake in a preheated 375 degree oven until firm and lightly browned—about 45 minutes. Let stand 5 minutes before cutting.

TO MICROWAVE: Roll pastry between 12-inch squares of waxed paper and line a 9-inch glass pie pan or quiche dish. Flute rim and prick the shell with a fork. Microwave on full power for 4½ minutes, turning once. Let stand to cool.

Chop onions by hand or in food processor. Combine with margarine and oil in a 1½-quart cooking dish. Cover and microwave on full power for 10 minutes, stirring once. Uncover and microwave for 5 minutes, stirring once. Set aside.

In food processor or mixing bowl, combine sour cream with skim milk powder, flour, salt and pepper. Chop cheese in half-inch chunks and add to processor, or shred and add to mixing bowl. Process or stir until blended. Add water and eggs and process or beat. Stir into cooked onions. Microwave, uncovered, for 4 minutes on full power, stirring once. Transfer to baked pastry shell and smooth top. Sprinkle with the 2 tablespoons of shredded cheese and the nutmeg. Microwave on full power for 2 minutes. Rotate one-third turn and microwave on half power (Defrost setting) for 8 minutes, turning one-third of the way around after 5 minutes. Let stand for 5 minutes before cutting.

SUPER-NUTRITION VARIATION:

Add with the flour: 1 ounce ALL STAR 95% PROTEIN
SUPREME powder
¼ teaspoon B-COMPLEX POWDER
¼ teaspoon C-TRATE

contents of 1 10,000 IU SUPER DRY
A & D capsule

Yield: 6 servings

SUNFLOWER-MILLET PATTIES

Sunflower seeds and millet are both excellent sources of essential nutrients in addition to those shown in the nutritional analysis tables (vitamin B_6, pantothenic acid, zinc, etc.) and combined in these patties offer an uncommonly good entree for meatless meals. Serve with mushroom or tomato sauce—or even use cold as a filling for pocket breads.

½ cup **SUNFLOWER SEED MEAL**

¼ cup non-instant **SKIM MILK POWDER**

¼ cup **WHEAT GERM**

¼ cup grated **Parmesan cheese**

½ teaspoon **SPIKE**

1 slice whole-wheat bread, crumbled

¼ large **green bell pepper,** minced

¼ medium **onion,** minced

1 large **egg**

2 tablespoons **ACIDOPHILUS YOGURT** (or buttermilk)

1 teaspoon **TAMARI SOY SAUCE**

¾ cup cooked **MILLET***

Combine sunflower seed meal, skim milk powder, wheat germ, grated cheese and Spike. Stir in crumbled bread, minced vegetables, egg, yogurt and soy sauce. When well blended, stir in millet.

WITH FOOD PROCESSOR: Sunflower seeds may be substituted for the meal and ground with the dry ingredients in the processor bowl. Add the crumbled bread and vegetables cut in chunks and process with cutting blade until finely minced. Add egg, yogurt and soy sauce and process 10 seconds. Add millet and process just enough to combine.

Shape into 4 patties. Fry until golden brown on both

---

*TO COOK DRY MILLET: Heat 1 cup of water with ⅛ teaspoon SEA SALT until boiling. Stir in ½ cup MILLET and continue stirring until mixture returns to boiling. Lower heat, cover tightly and simmer for 15 minutes—until all water is absorbed and grains are fluffy and tender.

sides on a lightly oiled griddle or preheated microwave browning grill.

SUPER-NUTRITION VARIATION:

- Add with the dry ingredients: 2 tablespoons LECITHIN GRANULES
  1 tablespoon BREWER'S YEAST
  contents of 1 10,000 IU SUPER DRY A & D capsule
  ⅛ teaspoon C-TRATE

Yield: 4 servings

VARIATION: *APPETIZER SUNFLOWER-MILLET BALLS*
Shape the mixture into ¾-inch balls, fry and drain on absorbent paper. Refrigerate or freeze until ready to serve, then re-heat on serving plate in the microwave oven, on a cookie sheet in the conventional oven, or on the tray of a toaster oven. Serve with picks and a tangy sauce for dunking.

Yield: 2 cups

TO MICROWAVE: Stir 3 tablespoons MILLET into ½ cup water in a 4-cup glass measure. Add ½ teaspoon OIL and a pinch of SEA SALT. Cover with a saucer and microwave on full power for 2 minutes, or until boiling. Set control on Defrost (half power) and microwave for 10 minutes. Let stand 5 minutes.

Yield: ¾ cup

SWISS POTATOES & ONIONS

The onions seem to disappear in this casserole spiced in such an intriguing way, leaving only a haunting flavor, plus their vitamins and minerals. With its lower carbohydrate count and high protein it is wonderful for vegetarian meals and appeals to today's "nouvelle cuisine" crusaders, yet is hearty enough to satisfy dedicated potato lovers.

2 medium onions
1 tablespoon COLD PRESSED ALL-BLEND OIL
1 tablespoon safflower margarine
4 medium potatoes (1 pound) peeled if desired
1 cup shredded natural Swiss cheese

⅓ cup non-instant SKIM MILK POWDER
1 tablespoon LECITHIN GRANULES
1 teaspoon SEA SALT
⅛ teaspoon ground black pepper
⅛ teaspoon ground mace
1 cup water
¼ teaspoon paprika

Quarter onions the long way and thinly slice by hand or with a food processor. Sauté with the oil and margarine until limp and just beginning to brown. Spoon half the onions into a 2-quart casserole.

Thinly slice potatoes, layer half of them over the onions and cover with half the shredded cheese.

Mix skim milk powder with lecithin granules, salt, pepper and mace in a small bowl. Gradually whisk in water and pour half the mixture over the layer of cheese in the casserole. Repeat layers of onions, potatoes and cheese. Pour remaining milk mixture over the top. Sprinkle with paprika, cover and bake in a preheated 350 degree oven for 45 minutes. Remove cover and continue baking until potatoes are tender and the top is crusty and brown—about 40 minutes.

TO MICROWAVE: Quarter onions the long way and thinly slice by hand or with a food processor. Combine with oil and margarine in a 1½-quart serving casserole. Cover and microwave on full power for 10 minutes, stirring after 5 minutes. Let stand, covered.

In a 2-quart cooking dish, combine skim milk powder with lecithin granules, salt, pepper and mace. Gradually whisk in water. Thinly slice the potatoes, by hand or with a food processor, and stir into the milk mixture. Cover and microwave on full power for 10 minutes—stirring halfway through the cooking time.

Add cheese to onions and stir in the boiling potatoes. Cover and microwave on full power for 5 minutes. Stir and smooth top. Dust with paprika, leave uncovered and microwave on full power until the potatoes are tender—about 6 minutes.

SUPER-NUTRITION VARIATION:

- Add with the salt: contents of one 5,000 IU SUPER DRY A & D capsule
  contents of one DAILY B-COMPLEX capsule
  ⅛ teaspoon C-TRATE

Yield: 4 servings

CHAPTER 5

Vegetables

DRIED BEANS & LEGUMES

FRESH VEGETABLES

DRIED BEANS & OTHER LEGUMES

Fortunately for our health, and our food budgets, dried legumes are back in the limelight as epicurean delights. A delicious example of serendipity, in addition to their healthful and economical attributes, beans are the easiest of all foods to store and prepare. Since beans develop in protective shells above the ground, they are the least likely of all our foods to be contaminated by harmful chemicals in the ground or in the air. Plain home-cooking enhances their flavor without any of the additives included in most canned products, and all types of cooked beans freeze well.

Nutritionally, beans are superb. As long as some whole grains, dairy products, nuts, corn or animal protein is included on the menu to compensate for the deficient amino acid in all beans except soys, they supply a complete protein—plus fiber, iron, magnesium, potassium, other minerals, and the B-complex vitamins.

Slow-cookers, pressure cookers and microwave ovens can tailor dried-bean cooking to fit any schedule but, when time permits, there is no way to improve on the soak-and-simmer method evolved by prehistoric cooks and followed since the Bronze Age. No more complex than boiling water, it is still the most effortless and economical way to cook beans in quantity for stocking the freezer.

Neither long soaking nor pre-cooking is actually necessary for any of the legumes except soybeans and garbanzos—but it does shorten cooking time and produce more tender-skinned beans that are easier to digest—especially when Instant Liquid Tenderizer is added.

BRONZE AGE BEANS

2 pounds (4 cups) any kind of dried beans except soys, which are dealt with on page 132

3 quarts water
1 teaspoon ALL BLEND OIL
1 tablespoon SEA SALT

Remove any foreign particles from the beans and rinse in a sieve under running water. Place in a 5-quart kettle with the water. Cover and let stand for 6 to 12 hours. Add oil and bring to boiling. Reduce heat, cover and simmer for 1 hour. Stir in salt, cover and continue simmering until tender—which can be anywhere from a few minutes longer for lima or pinto beans to 4 hours longer for garbanzos or black beans. Stir every half-hour or so and add a little hot liquid if the beans get too dry.

Ladle the 10 to 12 cups of cooked beans into small containers for quick freezing and brief defrosting. (If your freezer space is limited, reduce everything but the soaking and cooking times by one half.)

When the bean-cooking urge strikes without warning, you can forego the long soaking and resort to the PRE-COOK METHOD:

Add the teaspoon of oil to the rinsed beans and water. Add 1 teaspoon INSTANT LIQUID TENDERIZER and let stand for 5 minutes. Bring to a full boil for 2 minutes. Remove from heat, cover and let stand for 1 hour, then cook as for the long-soaked beans.

Twentieth-century appliances do have their advantages over more primitive methods. One pound of beans, either soaked or pre-cooked, can be salted and left to fend for itself all day in a slow-cooker. (If you haven't cooked dry beans in your slow-cooker, experiment with the first pound when you are at home to check on it—some brands of cookers require occasional stirring to prevent over-done beans on the bottom and underdone ones in the center.) With a large pressure cooker you can put the pound of beans to soak in the morning and cook them in half-an-hour after your return in the evening. (Amounts and cooking times vary with individual cookers, but they all produce beautifully plump and tender beans.) For the days when life is real and

earnest and thoughts of dinner don't surface until 5 p.m. . . . . and
you'd really like to have some beans but there aren't any cooked
ones on hand . . . Instant Liquid Tenderizer and a small pressure
cooker or a microwave oven can come to the rescue.

QUICK METHOD FOR SMALL PRESSURE COOKERS: Most pressure cookers may be half filled with beans and liquid, but some brands limit the quantity to one-third—1 to 1½ cups of dried beans cook perfectly in the 2½ to 3-quart electric pressure cookers. Allow 25 minutes for lima beans; 30 minutes for red, white or brown beans; and 40 minutes for soys, garbanzos or black beans.)

1 cup (½ pound dry beans)	1 tablespoon COLD
3 cups hot tap water	PRESSED ALL BLEND
1 teaspoon INSTANT	OIL
LIQUID TENDERIZER	1 teaspoon SEA SALT

    Place the washed beans in the pressure cooker with water, tenderizer and oil and let stand for 5 minutes. (The extra oil prevents foaming that could clog the vent pipe.) Bring to boiling in the open pressure cooker. Turn off, or remove from the heat source. Cover and let stand for 1 hour. Stir in the salt and add water if needed to cover the beans. Close cover securely and put pressure control in place. When pressure is reached, cook for the 25 to 40 minutes and let the pressure drop of its own accord.

Yield: 2½ to 3 cups cooked beans

QUICK METHOD FOR MICROWAVE OVENS: One pound of dried beans can be microwaved in a 5-quart casserole, but for quantity cooking, a large pressure cooker is faster. Four servings do microwave quickly and offer the advantages of requiring only the one cook-and-serve casserole, being able to add seasonings or other ingredients during cooking, and never producing mushy beans—overcooking merely dries the outer layer.

⅔ cup dried beans	1 teaspoon COLD
2½ cups hot tap water	PRESSED ALL BLEND
1 teaspoon INSTANT	OIL
LIQUID TENDERIZER	½ teaspoon SEA SALT

Place washed beans in a 2-quart casserole with the water, tenderizer and oil. Let stand for 5 minutes. Cover and microwave on full power for 6 minutes, or until the beans are boiling. Let stand for 1 hour. Stir, cover and microwave on full power until boiling— about 5 minutes. Set control on Defrost (half power) and microwave, covered, for 20 minutes. Stir in salt, cover and continue microwaving on half power until the beans are tender— adding a little hot water if the beans become too dry. Depending on the variety and age of the beans, this last cooking period will require 10 to 30 minutes.

Yield: Approximately 2 cups cooked beans

GENERAL COOKING NOTES:

● The minerals in hard water may prevent dried beans from softening, no matter how long they are cooked. You can counteract this by adding a small amount of baking soda to the cooking water, but never use more than ¼ teaspoon of soda for each pound of dried beans or some of the B vitamins will be destroyed.

● When cooking garbanzos or soy beans, substituting COLD PRESSED SESAME OIL for the All Blend Oil adds a sprightly, nut-like flavor.

● For added flavor and food value, beef, chicken or vegetable broth may be substituted for water as the cooking liquid. (Refrigerate the beans and broth if using the long-soaking method.)

● Unless using a pressure cooker or slow-cooker, the salt and wine or other acidic liquids should not be added until the beans are partially cooked to avoid toughening the beans. Interrupting the cooking process also causes tough beans—add only hot liquids or ingredients while the beans are cooking.

TWENTIETH CENTURY BAKED BEANS

A supply of cooked beans guarantees a multitude of ready-when-you-are menus. The 1930s depression fare of beans ladled over a slice of homemade bread was nutritious but is a bit austere for current lifestyles. Colonial New England's Sunday meal of baked beans and brown bread, however, requires only a salad and dessert to bring it up-to-date, and modern cooking methods need only 10 to 30 minutes to duplicate the 24 hour baking.

2 cups cooked navy, great north-ern or pea beans plus ⅓ to ½ cup of the cooking liquid
1½ teaspoons ARROWROOT or cornstarch
½ teaspoon dry mustard
¼ teaspoon SEA SALT
⅛ teaspoon ground white pepper
⅛ teaspoon C-TRATE
¼ cup tomato juice

2 tablespoons Instant Ketchup (recipe on page 156)
1 tablespoon APPLE CIDER VINEGAR
1 tablespoon PURE MAPLE SYRUP
1 tablespoon BLACKSTRAP MOLASSES
1 tablespoon minced onion

Place beans and cooking liquid in a 1-quart, flame-proof casserole over low heat. In a small bowl, combine arrow-root, mustard, salt, pepper and C-Trate. Gradually add tomato juice, stirring to keep smooth. Add ketchup, vine-gar, maple syrup, molasses and minced onion and stir into the beans. Cook and stir until boiling. Cover and bake in a preheated 375 degree oven for 20 minutes, uncovering during the last 10 minutes.

TO MICROWAVE: Place beans and ⅓ cup of their cooking liquid in a 1-quart cooking-serving dish and microwave on full power until simmering—2 to 5 minutes, depending on their starting temperature. In a small bowl, combine arrowroot, mustard, salt, pepper and C-Trate. Gradually add tomato juice, stirring to keep smooth. Add remaining ingredients and stir into the beans. Microwave, uncovered, on full power for 8 minutes, stirring after 4 minutes.

Yield: 4 servings

SUPER-NUTRITION VARIATION # 1:

* Add with the dry mustard: ¼ teaspoon VITAMIN B-COMPLEX POWDER contents of 1 5,000 IU SUPER DRY A & D capsule

SUPER-NUTRITION VARIATION # 2:
TWENTIETH CENTURY BAKED SOYBEANS

Substitute cooked soybeans and their liquid for all or part of the white beans.

BEANS WITH FRUIT

Combining fruit with beans gives a new dimension to bean dishes. The bits of fruit add lightness plus tantalizing new flavors, as well as vitamins, minerals and fiber to our already nutritious beans. Fresh or frozen fruit lends excitement to cold bean salads (see Tropical Garbanzo Salad on page 40) and evokes visions of Latin America and the tropics in spicy hot dishes.

BAKED KIDNEY BEANS WITH PEARS

2 tablespoons RAW BROWN SUGAR
1 teaspoon ARROWROOT or cornstarch
¾ teaspoon dry mustard
½ teaspoon chili powder
¼ teaspoon SEA SALT

1¼ cups cooked, drained kidney beans plus ⅓ to ½ cup cooking liquid
1 tablespoon APPLE CIDER VINEGAR
1 large, ripe pear (6 ounces)

In a 1-quart, flame-proof casserole combine brown sugar, arrowroot, mustard, chili powder and salt. Stir in bean cooking liquid and vinegar. Cook and stir until boiling. Stir in beans. Core pear, remove peeling only if coarse or blemished, and cut into pieces approximately the same size as the beans. Stir in, cover and bake in a preheated, 350 degree oven for 30 minutes, uncovering during the final 10 minutes.

TO MICROWAVE: Combine dry ingredients in a 1-quart cooking-serving dish. Stir in bean cooking liquid and vinegar. Microwave, uncovered, for 3 minutes on full power, stirring once. Stir in beans and cored, diced pear. Cover and microwave on full power for 3 minutes. Stir, leave uncovered and microwave for 3 minutes on full power.

SUPER-NUTRITION VARIATION:

- Use only 1 tablespoon raw brown sugar
- Add with the dry ingredients:
  ¼ teaspoon C-TRATE
  contents of 1 DAILY B-COMPLEX capsule
  contents of 1 5,000 IU SUPER DRY A & D capsule
- Add 1 tablespoon BLACKSTRAP MOLASSES with the cooking liquid and vinegar

Yield: 4 servings

SWEET & SOUR BEANS

An uncommonly good bean dish, worthy of entree status on a vegetarian menu.

1 teaspoon COLD PRESSED PEANUT OIL	2 tablespoons ARROWROOT or cornstarch
1 medium onion, quartered and thinly sliced to make slivers	½ teaspoon SEA SALT
1 medium green bell pepper in ½-inch squares	⅛ teaspoon ground white pepper
¼ cup RAW BROWN SUGAR	⅛ teaspoon garlic powder
	2 cups cooked, drained small red beans*

---

*Swedish brown beans or kidney beans may be substituted.

⅓ cup cooking liquid from beans	½ teaspoon TAMARI SOY SAUCE
2 slices canned pineapple, juice pack, plus ⅓ cup of the liquid	2 tablespoons chopped pimiento
3 tablespoons APPLE CIDER VINEGAR	¼ teaspoon C-TRATE
	contents of 1 5,000 IU SUPER DRY A & D capsule (optional)

Sauté onion and bell pepper until limp but not browned in the peanut oil. Combine in a small saucepan the brown sugar, arrowroot, salt, white pepper and garlic powder. Stir in bean cooking liquid, pineapple juice and vinegar. Cook and stir until thickened and beginning to boil. Stir in soy sauce, beans, pineapple, pimiento, C-Trate, and the contents of the A & D capsule, if used. Heat to serving temperature.

TO MICROWAVE: Combine onion, pepper and oil in a 1-quart cooking-serving dish. Microwave on full power, uncovered, for 3 minutes—stirring once.

In a 2-cup glass measure, combine the sugar, arrowroot, salt, white pepper and garlic. Stir in pineapple juice, cooking liquid from beans and vinegar. Microwave, uncovered, for 4 minutes on full power, stirring after 2 minutes. Stir into onion-pepper mixture with soy sauce, beans, pineapple, pimiento, C-Trate and the contents of the A & D capsule, if used. Microwave, uncovered, just to serving temperature—stirring once if beans were cold.

Yield: 4 servings

GOLDEN DELICIOUS LIMAS

Another example of unexpected combinations proving to be unexpectedly delicious. The onions and apples melt into the background to give the limas a light and zestful taste and texture. They also add their vitamins and minerals to the beans' prodigious amounts of potassium (5 milligrams per bean), iron, fiber, B vitamins and zinc.

1 tablespoon safflower margarine
½ medium onion, chopped
2 tablespoons RAW BROWN SUGAR, firmly packed
1 teaspoon dry mustard
½ teaspoon SEA SALT
¼ teaspoon B-COMPLEX POWDER (optional)
¼ teaspoon C-TRATE

1 5,000 IU SUPER DRY A & D capsule (optional)
2 Golden Delicious apples (1½ cups chopped) 6 ounces
2 cups cooked, drained, large lima beans
⅛ teaspoon freshly ground black pepper

Heat margarine in a skillet and sauté onion until limp but not browned. Remove from heat and stir in brown sugar, dry mustard, salt, B-complex powder and the contents of the A & D capsule (if used) with the vitamin C powder. Wash and core apples but peel only if skins are blemished or tough. Chop and stir into the onion mixture. Cover and cook over low heat, stirring frequently, until apples are almost tender—about 10 minutes. Stir in lima beans and black pepper and heat to serving temperature.

TO MICROWAVE: Cut margarine in quarters and microwave with the onions for 3 minutes, uncovered, on full power—stirring after 2 minutes. Stir in brown sugar, mustard, salt, B-complex powder and the contents of the A & D capsule (if used) with the vitamin C powder. Wash and core apples but peel only if skins are blemished or tough. Chop and stir into the onion mixture. Cover and microwave on full power for 5 minutes, stirring after 3 minutes. Stir in lima beans and black pepper and heat to serving temperature.

Yield: 4 servings

SOYS, THE MAGIC BEANS

Excelling even the fabled beans of Jack and the Beanstalk, soybeans grow tall people instead of vines. (Their use in the provinces of northern China is said to be the reason that northern Chinese are taller than southern Chinese.) The magic lies in their high percentage of complete protein, low carbohydrate content, and complete range of vitamins and minerals which not only affect growth but provide energy and good health. Even the fat in soybeans is beneficial as it consists of unsaturated fatty acids and contains lecithin.

Soybeans are available in many forms: chopped into small bits for Soy Grits or Granules to cook with cereals or use as a meat extender; ground into a flour so full of nourishment it is used as a food supplement; pressed to make soybean oil; or transformed into Lecithin Liquid, Granules or Powder. Dry soybeans can be sprouted to acquire vitamin C and increase the vitamin A content (the sprouts may be eaten raw but the beans and raw flour should be cooked in order to nullify the anti-enzyme factor which would otherwise interfere with trypsin, a necessary digestive enzyme), and either soy flour or beans can be used to make soymilk.

Dried soybeans need a little more cooking time to become tender than do other dried beans. Either soaking the washed beans for 24 hours in the refrigerator or letting them stand for two hours after coming to a boil for the pre-cook method will shorten the cooking time, and Instant Liquid Tenderizer assists in the tenderizing.

TO COOK DRY SOYBEANS

2 cups dry YELLOW SOYBEANS

7 cups water (using part beef, chicken or vegetable broth adds flavor)

2 teaspoons INSTANT LIQUID TENDERIZER

1 tablespoon COLD PRESSED SESAME OIL

1 teaspoon SEA SALT

LONG SOAKING METHOD: Wash the beans under running water. Combine with liquid and soak for 12 to 24 hours. (Refrigerating the beans and liquid avoids any possibility of souring.)

PRE-COOK METHOD: Combine the washed beans with liquid, tenderizer and oil. Let stand for 10 minutes and bring to boiling. Remove from heat, cover and let stand for 1½ to 2 hours.

Stove-top Soybeans: Add tenderizer and oil (if not used in pre-cooking) and bring to a boil. Reduce heat and simmer over low heat until almost tender before adding salt. Continue simmering until tender.

Slow-cooker Soybeans: Combine soaked or pre-cooked soybeans with tenderizer, oil and salt. Cover and cook on Low until tender, stirring once or twice if convenient, and testing after 12 hours. Soybeans can take from 12 to 16 hours to cook.

Pressure cooking and microwaving require approximately the same amount of elapsed time. A larger quantity can be cooked at one time in a 4 or 6 quart pressure cooker and the beans are melt-in-your-mouth tender. Microwaved soybeans have a little more character even when well done and are ideal for bean salads or stir-fry dishes.

Pressure Cooker Soybeans: Follow the manufacturer's instructions for the amount of beans, water and oil to use with your cooker. Soak the washed beans for at least 12 hours or pre-cook with tenderizer and oil and let stand for 1½ to 2 hours. Stir in salt, cover and put pressure control in place. Cook for 40 minutes after full pressure is reached and allow the pressure to drop normally.

Microwaved Soybeans: ⅔ cup dry YELLOW SOYBEANS
2 cups water
½ teaspoon INSTANT LIQUID TENDERIZER
2 teaspoons COLD PRESSED SESAME OIL
½ teaspoon SEA SALT

Combine washed soybeans, water, tenderizer and sesame oil in a 2-quart casserole and let stand 10 minutes. Cover and microwave on full power until boiling—about 6 minutes. Let stand for 1½ to 2 hours.

Microwave covered, on full power, until boiling—about 5 minutes. Stir, cover and microwave on Defrost (half power) for 30 minutes. Stir in salt, cover and microwave on Defrost for another 30 minutes—or until as tender as desired.

Yield: 1⅔ to 2 cups cooked, drained beans

Cooked soybeans are quite bland and can be incorporated with other beans when making chili con carne and/or other highly spiced dishes, served with any well-flavored sauce (see Baked Soybeans, page 127), or substituted for other cooked beans in combination dishes. However they are served, the magical soybean can become a nutritious and economical addition to our diets as shown by the following comparison chart.

BEAN COMPARISON CHART*

per 100 grams dry beans (approximately ½ cup)	White Beans	Pinto, Calico & Red Beans	Lima Beans	Soybeans
Calories	340	349	345	403
Protein, g	22.3 (inc)	22.9 (inc)	20.4 (inc)	34.1 (complete)
Fat, g	1.6	1.2	1.6	17.7
Carbohydrate, g	61.3	63.7	64.0	33.5
Fiber, g	4.3	4.3	4.3	4.9
Calcium, mg	144.0	135.0	72.0	226.0
Iron, mg	7.8	6.4	7.8	8.4
Potassium, mg	1196.0	984.0	1529.0	1677.0
Vitamin B_1, mg	.65	.84	.48	1.1
Vitamin B_2, mg	.22	.21	.17	.3
Niacin, mg	2.4	2.2	1.9	2.2

*from USDA Handbook #8.

SOY SUCCOTASH

Soybeans can be substituted for limas in standard succotash, but for a quickly prepared, unusually flavorful combination, try this "fried" version as either a side dish with a meal light in protein, or as a vegetarian entree.

1 tablespoon COLD
   PRESSED ALL BLEND
   OIL
1 medium onion, quartered and
   thinly sliced to make slivers
1 cup frozen corn, defrosted
   enough to separate

1 cup cooked, drained
   SOYBEANS
¼ cup soybean cooking
   liquid
1 teaspoon SPIKE
¼ cup (1 ounce) shredded
   sharp natural cheddar
   cheese

Sauté onion in oil until limp but not browned. Stir in corn, soybeans, cooking liquid and Spike. Cover and simmer over low heat for 10 minutes. Transfer to serving dish or individual plates and sprinkle with cheese.

> **TO MICROWAVE:** Combine oil and onion in a 1-quart casserole. Cover and microwave for 3 minutes. Stir in corn, soybeans, cooking liquid and Spike. Cover and microwave for 3 minutes. Stir, leave uncovered and microwave for 3 minutes. Sprinkle with cheese and let stand 1 minute before serving.

Yield: 4 servings

SOYMILK

Soymilk is easily prepared from soy flour or dried soy beans, and provides a bonus of meat-extender.

SOYMILK #1, made with soy flour
1 cup SOY FLOUR
4 cups water

Gradually stir the water into the flour in the top of a double boiler. Cover and let stand for 2 hours. Place the mixture over boiling water, stir, cover and cook for 30 minutes—or until the temperature reaches 150 degrees.

TO MICROWAVE: Combine flour and water in a 2-quart casserole. Cover and let stand for 2 hours. Stir, cover and microwave on full power for 4 minutes. Turn dish, set control on Defrost (half power) and microwave for 8 minutes—or until the temperature reaches 150 degrees.

Strain through a sieve with 1/16-inch mesh and let cool before storing in the refrigerator. (The residue remaining in the sieve may be added to a meatloaf or casserole to utilize all the nutrients.)

Yield: 1 quart soymilk

SOYMILK #2 PLUS MEAT EXTENDER, made with dry soybeans

1 cup dry YELLOW SOYBEANS
6 cups water, divided

Wash beans and place in a saucepan with 4 cups of the water. Cover and let stand 10 to 12 hours. Heat to boiling, reduce heat and simmer, covered, for 15 minutes.

TO MICROWAVE: Soak the washed beans in a 2-quart casserole with 4 cups of water for 10 to 12 hours. Microwave on full power until boiling—about 8 minutes—then set on Defrost (half power) and microwave, covered, for 8 minutes.

Add 2 cups of cold water and grind the mixture one half at a time in an electric blender on medium speed. Strain through a sieve with 1/16-inch mesh; stir with a spoon to speed the draining but do not rub the pulp through the sieve. Reserve the pulp and rinse the sieve, then strain the milk a second time without stirring—to remove the last of the ground beans.

Store the milk in a freshly washed glass bottle in the refrigerator. Place the pulp in a covered container and refrigerate. This pulp may be added to casseroles or to the batter for muffins or waffles, or used as a meat extender.

MEAT EXTENDER: Mix ½ cup of the pulp with each ¾ pound of raw ground beef, chicken or pork; then use as 1 pound of ground meat in recipes. (Soy meat extender can also be prepared from soy grits or granules as in the recipe for Sunflower-Mushroom Meatloaf on page 70.)

Yield: 1 quart soymilk plus 2 1/3 cups meat-extender pulp

SOYMILK AS A BEVERAGE: For those who cannot tolerate milk, soymilk can be made a palatable beverage by adding a teaspoon of RAW HONEY and a pinch of SEA SALT to each quart. (Powdered DOLOMITE and BONE MEAL may be added for extra calcium.)

ENRICHED SOYMILK

Fortifying soymilk with supplements plus non-instant skim milk powder can provide a real nutrition booster in beverages and recipes calling for fluid milk—note the comparison chart below.

1 quart soymilk
⅓ cup non-instant SKIM MILK POWDER
¼ teaspoon DOLOMITE POWDER
¼ teaspoon BONE MEAL POWDER
1 5,000 IU SUPER DRY A & D capsule

Pour 1 cup of the soymilk into the container of an electric blender. Add skim milk powder, dolomite, bone meal and the contents of the A & D capsule. Blend on high speed until smooth. (Or beat with an eggbeater in a mixing bowl.) Add remaining soymilk and blend on low speed. Store in the refrigerator in a covered bottle.

COMPARISON CHART

	Fortified Fluid Skim Milk*	Fresh Whole Milk*	Soymilk*	Enriched Soymilk (above)
per cup				
Calories	86.	159.	75.	113.
Protein, grams	8.35	8.5	7.7	11.57
Fat, grams	.44	8.15	3.4	3.5
Carbohydrates, grams	11.8	11.4	5.1	8.9
Calcium, milligrams	302.	291.	47.5	309.
Vitamin A, International Units	500.	350.	90.	1345.
Vitamin B₁, milligrams	.08	.09	.18	.22
Niacin, milligrams	.21	.20	.50	.56

*from *Nutrition Almanac*, McGraw Hill Paperback, New York 1979

FRESH VEGETABLES

To rate gourmet classification, foods need be neither exotic nor elaborate, and this is especially true of vegetables. Simply steamed, dressed with a bit of safflower margarine or "healthy butter" (page 151) and a touch of seasoning, vegetables offer a rainbow of color to make each meal a masterpiece. Altering the traditional shapes of vegetables adds visual appeal to otherwise familiar fare, and varying the vegetable combinations creates the excitement of new and different taste sensations. Fresh herbs have an almost magical alchemy with vegetables, transforming even everyday carrots, celery and zucchini into savory spectaculars. (Fresh herbs are sometimes available from the produce counter, but the best way to be assured a constant supply is to grow your own—they make attractive houseplants.)

Some vitamin loss occurs with the storage and preparation of most vegetables but this can be kept to a minimum by chilling them before slicing or chopping; never soaking them in water; and using all of the cooking liquid—either in the dish being prepared or in soups—as it contains most of the water-soluble nutrients. Vitamin C powder (C-TRATE) is heat stable, so it may be added to replace what is destroyed by cooking.

A microwave oven is a kitchen magician when it comes to steaming vegetables. Whole cauliflower is a show-stopper when snugly wrapped in plastic, microwaved for 10 minutes, then unwrapped and showered with shredded cheese. Peas, carrots, cut corn, etc., steam to perfection when microwaved in a tightly covered serving bowl with 1 teaspoon each water and margarine. Cabbage microwaves beautifully in eight minutes when the wedges are arranged spoke-fashion in a pie plate and tightly covered with plastic.

"Pretty as a picture" vegetable platters can serve as dinner centerpieces and are subject to unlimited artistry. The easiest and most strikingly effective arrangement is a series of concentric circles of zucchini slices, green pepper rings, sliced mushrooms, broccoli or cauliflower florets, tiny boiling onions, cherry tomatoes, etc., with the quickest-cooking vegetables placed in the center. For tender carrots or green beans, microwave with a teaspoon of water and a teaspoon of margarine in a small covered container for about 5 minutes before adding to the platter. The center may be reserved for a small bowl of separately heated sauce, or for a small partially cooked head of cauliflower. When the design is complete, cover the entire platter with plastic wrap, tucking the edges under the plate for double security, and microwave on full power until the vegetables are as tender-crunchy as desired. This can take from 5 to 15 minutes, depending on the vegetables and amounts, and the platter should be rotated one-quarter turn several times for even cooking.

In addition to providing beauty without bother, this form of steaming intensifies the flavors so that very little salt or seasoning is required, and preserves all of the nutrients since none are dissipated in aromatic steam or cooking water.

HERBED CARROTS

¼ cup water
¼ teaspoon LIQUID FRUCTOSE
¾ pound carrots
1 tablespoon safflower margarine
1 tablespoon Marsala wine or apple juice
1 tablespoon snipped fresh basil*
¼ teaspoon SEA SALT
⅛ teaspoon C-TRATE
⅛ teaspoon freshly ground black pepper

Combine water and fructose in a heavy-bottomed saucepan, cover and bring to boiling. Scrape or peel carrots and slice. Stir into boiling water with margarine and wine. Cover and cook until carrots are as tender as desired, 15 to 20 minutes, stirring occasionally. Stir in basil and cook, uncovered, until most of the liquid has evaporated. Stir in salt, C-Trate and pepper.

TO MICROWAVE: Reduce water to 2 tablespoons. Combine water, fructose and wine in a 1½-quart casserole. Stir in peeled, sliced carrots. Add margarine, cover and microwave on full power for 12 minutes, stirring after 6 minutes. Stir in basil and microwave for a minute or so, if necessary, to evapo-

*Dill, mint, oregano, parsley, savory or any favorite herb may be used in place of the basil. To substitute dry herbs, refresh 1 teaspoon of the crushed, dried herb by mixing it with an additional teaspoon of wine and letting the mixture stand for 15 minutes. Add to the carrots as directed.

rate excess liquid. Sprinkle with salt, C-Trate and pepper.

Yield: 4 servings

SPRING SKILLET—CARROTS AND SCALLIONS

When cut into long, thin slices, even winter carrots have spring-time freshness accentuated by the fresh green of onions and parsley.

½ pound carrots, as small as available

2 tablespoons chicken broth, homemade or canned

1 tablespoon safflower margarine

1 large bunch green onions with crisp tops

¾ teaspoon SPIKE

2 tablespoons snipped parsley

⅛ teaspoon C-TRATE

Peel or scrape carrots and cut in lengthwise halves or quarters if more than ½-inch in diameter. Slice with a vegetable peeler into long, wafer-thin strips and place in a sauté pan or medium skillet. Add broth and margarine. Cover and bring to a full boil over medium heat.

Wash onions and trim to 5 or 6-inch lengths. Slice in lengthwise halves or quarters unless very tiny. Stir into carrots and sprinkle with Spike. Cover and return to boiling, then uncover and stir constantly until tender-crisp—about 5 minutes—being careful not to allow the vegetables to brown. Sprinkle with parsley and C-Trate and stir-fry for another minute.

TO MICROWAVE: Prepare carrots as for conventional cooking, then combine with broth and margarine in a shallow, 1-quart casserole. Microwave on full power, covered, for 3 minutes. Prepare onions as directed and stir into the mixture. Sprinkle with Spike, cover and microwave for 3 minutes. Stir in parsley and C-Trate, cover and microwave for 1 minute.

Yield: 4 servings

MINTED CELERY

¼ cup chicken broth, homemade or canned

3 cups celery in 1-inch diagonal slices

½ cup chopped onion

1 tablespoon safflower margarine

2 tablespoons chopped fresh mint leaves

½ teaspoon SPIKE

⅛ teaspoon C-TRATE

Bring the broth to boiling in a small, heavy-bottomed saucepan. Wash and trim celery. Finely chop ½ cup of the leaves and include with the 3 cups of sliced celery. Stir into the broth with the onion. Add margarine, cover and steam for 10 minutes. Stir in mint, Spike and C-Trate. Cover and return to the heat until as tender as desired—1 minute for crisp-tender, longer for well done.

TO MICROWAVE: Pour broth into a 1-quart casserole. Wash and trim celery. Finely chop ½ cup of the leaves and include to make the 3 cups of sliced celery. Stir into the broth with the onion. Add margarine, cover and microwave on full power for 4 minutes. Stir in mint, Spike and C-Trate. Cover and microwave 1 minute for crisp-tender celery, 3 minutes for well done.

Yield: 4 servings

CORN CAKES

¼ cup Seasoned Flour (recipe on page 154)

1 tablespoon SOY FLOUR

1 tablespoon LECITHIN GRANULES

1 tablespoon non-instant SKIM MILK POWDER

¼ teaspoon chili powder

¼ teaspoon SEA SALT

½ medium onion

½ large green bell pepper

⅔ cup frozen, whole kernel corn, defrosted enough to separate

1 large egg

1 tablespoon COLD PRESSED PEANUT OIL

Combine Seasoned Flour, soy flour, lecithin, skim milk powder, chili powder and salt in a mixing bowl. Finely chop onion and green pepper. Stir in with corn and slightly beaten egg.

WITH FOOD PROCESSOR: In work bowl with cutting blade, place Seasoned Flour, soy flour, lecithin granules, skim milk powder, chili powder and salt. Process for 3 on/off turns or pulsations. Cut onion and pepper in chunks and process for 5 pulsations. Add corn and egg and process for 5 pulsations.

Spoon onto heated oil in a skillet or preheated microwave browning dish. Fry until golden brown on both sides.

Yield: 4 large or 6 medium corn cakes

CUCUMBER-ONION STIR FRY

1 tablespoon COLD PRESSED PEANUT OIL
1 large onion, quartered and sliced to make shreds (6 ounces)
1 large cucumber (6 ounces)
1 teaspoon SPIKE
¼ teaspoon C-TRATE

1 5,000 IU SUPER DRY A & D capsule (optional)
¼ cup Tropical Dressing (recipe on page 30)
½ teaspoon TAMARI SOY SAUCE

Sauté onion in oil until limp but not browned. Wash and dry cucumber, remove ends and blemishes but do not peel. Cut in half lengthwise and thinly slice. Stir into onion, cover and cook over low heat—stirring frequently—until crisp tender, about 10 minutes. Sprinkle with Spike, C-Trate and the contents of the A & D capsule (if used). Stir in Tropical Dressing and soy sauce. Cook and stir, uncovered, until most of the liquid has evaporated.

TO MICROWAVE: Combine oil and onion in a 1-quart cooking-serving dish. Microwave, uncovered, for 2 minutes on full power. Wash and dry cucumber, remove ends and blemishes but do not peel. Cut in half lengthwise and thinly slice. Stir into onion, cover and microwave on full power for 5 minutes—stirring after 3 minutes. (If not as tender as desired, microwave for an additional minute.) Stir in remaining ingredients, cover and microwave 2 minutes on full power. Stir and microwave for 2 minutes on full power, without covering so the excess liquid can evaporate.

Yield: 4 servings

PARSNIP PATTIES

Light and tender, these patties offer parsnips at their best—with their flavor, fiber and vitamins bolstered with extra protein from the milk, soy flour and egg.

¾ pound parsnips
⅓ cup water
2 tablespoons non-instant SKIM MILK POWDER
1 tablespoon SOY FLOUR
¼ teaspoon SEA SALT
1 large egg
1 tablespoon COLD PRESSED PEANUT OIL

Peel or scrape parsnips and cut into ¼-inch crosswise slices. Bring water to boiling in a saucepan. Add parsnips, cover and cook until tender—about 15 minutes. (Or microwave parsnips and water in a covered bowl for 8 minutes.) Let parsnips stand, covered, for 5 minutes.

Combine skim milk powder, soy flour and sea salt in processor or electric mixer bowl. Pour in cooking liquid from parsnips, stirring to keep smooth. Add parsnips and egg and process or beat until smooth.

Oil hot griddle or preheated microwave browning dish with peanut oil. Spoon on parsnip mixture to make four large or eight small patties and cook until golden brown on both sides.

Yield: 4 servings

SCALLOPED POTATOES

A quick and easy method of duplicating the old-fashioned flavor of potatoes layered with flour, butter, seasonings and milk. The "cooked in taste" is the same but less flour and fat is required.

¼ cup Seasoned Flour (recipe on page 154)

¼ cup non-instant SKIM MILK POWDER

¼ teaspoon SEA SALT

1 cup water

3½ cups sliced, peeled potatoes (1¼ pounds before peeling)

1 tablespoon snipped fresh parsley

1 tablespoon safflower margarine

In 2½-quart casserole, combine flour, dry milk and salt. Gradually stir in water. Mix in sliced potatoes and parsley. Cut margarine in quarters and dot over the surface. Cover and bake in a preheated, 350 degree oven for 45 minutes. Remove cover and continue baking until potatoes are tender and the top is slightly browned—about 15 minutes longer.

TO MICROWAVE: Prepare as directed. Cover and microwave on full power for 5 minutes. Stir, set control on half power (Defrost setting), cover and microwave for 8 minutes. If the potatoes are not quite tender, microwave, uncovered, for 3 to 5 minutes on full power. Dust with paprika or dry Rotisserie Magic (recipe on page 155) to compensate for the lack of a browned crust; or lightly brown with a microwave browner or under a conventional broiler if the potatoes are in a suitable container.

NOTE: Using a teflon-lined casserole for conventional baking saves having a sticky dish to clean— microwaved foods won't stick unless browned conventionally.

Yield: 4 servings

STUFFED BAKED POTATOES

Potatoes are naturally well-endowed with vitamins and minerals. With the addition of cottage cheese and vitamin C powder, they are even more nutritious, taste as luxurious as the usual sour cream-topped potatoes, and provide more protein with fewer calories.

4 medium or 2 large baking potatoes (1¼ pounds)	⅓ cup creamed, small-curd cottage cheese
1 tablespoon safflower margarine	¼ teaspoon SEA SALT
2 medium sized green onions, with crisp tops	¼ teaspoon C-TRATE
	paprika

Bake potatoes in either conventional or microwave oven and let stand for 10 minutes, covered.

While potatoes are standing, thinly slice onions and sauté in margarine until limp but not browned. Stir in cottage cheese to heat through. Transfer to mixing bowl. Cut potatoes in half, lengthwise, and scoop potato into the mixing bowl. Mash by hand or beat with an electric mixer until fluffy. Beat in salt and C-Trate.

WITH MICROWAVE OVEN AND FOOD PROCESSOR: Thinly slice onions and place in a glass measuring cup with the margarine. Microwave on full power for 1 minute. Stir in cottage cheese and microwave 1 more minute on full power. Transfer to processor bowl with cutting blade in place. Cut potatoes in half, lengthwise, and scoop into processor. Add salt and C-Trate and process just until smooth.

Pile into potato shells and reheat briefly, if necessary. Dust with paprika. May be prepared ahead of time and refrigerated or frozen.

Yield: 4 servings

YAM & PEANUT BOATS

An exciting, different (and nutritious) change from the usual candied yams; the flavor of the peanuts is subtle enough to enchant young and old alike and the carotene (vegetable vitamin A) is in its most assimilable form. When the lovely red yams are plentiful, prepare a fleet of Yam Boats, freeze them on a cookie sheet, then store in a plastic bag. Defrost and heat to serving temperature in either a conventional or microwave oven.

2 medium sized yams or sweet potatoes (1¼ pounds)	3 tablespoons NATURAL PEANUT BUTTER
¼ cup raw or dry-roasted peanuts, chopped	1 tablespoon safflower margarine
¼ cup milk	½ teaspoon KELP SEASONING
	¼ teaspoon SEA SALT

Wash potatoes and bake in a preheated 350 degree oven for 45 minutes, or until tender. Chop peanuts by hand or in a processor or blender and reserve.

Heat milk, peanut butter, margarine, kelp seasoning and salt in a small saucepan and pour into a mixing bowl or the bowl of a food processor.

Cut yams in half, lengthwise, and scoop centers into the peanut butter mixture. Mash, process or beat until smooth. Pile into the potato shells and sprinkle with the chopped peanuts, pressing gently to make them adhere. Reheat to serving temperature in the oven.

TO MICROWAVE: Scrub yams, pierce with the tip of a sharp knife and microwave on a paper towel for 7 minutes on full power. (Potatoes should feel slightly soft.) Wrap in the paper towel and let stand for 5 minutes.

Microwave milk, peanut butter, margarine, kelp seasoning and salt in a mixing bowl or in a glass measuring cup for 1½ minutes on full power. Pour into the work bowl of a food processor if it is to be used. Cut yams in half, lengthwise, and scoop centers into the peanut butter mixture. Mash, process or beat until smooth. Pile into the potato shells and sprinkle with the chopped peanuts, gently pressing to make them adhere. Reheat to serving temperature in the microwave oven.

Yield: 4 servings

CHAPTER 6

Condiments, Sauces & Syrups

BUTTERS

Add polyunsaturates, vitamin E and lecithin to your butter or safflower margarine for use as a table spread, for seasoning vegetables, or for sautéeing. (Neither the nutritional composition nor the total yield of these butters can be given because of the variance in margarines and butters and in the volume increase from processing or beating.)

"HEALTHY BUTTER"

1 cup room-temperature safflower margarine or butter (2 ¼-pound sticks)
⅓ cup COLD PRESSED SAFFLOWER OIL

2 tablespoons COLD PRESSED WHEAT GERM OIL
1 teaspoon LIQUID LECITHIN

Place all ingredients in a mixing bowl or in a food processor work bowl and beat or process until smooth and creamy. Store in the refrigerator in 1-cup covered serving bowls or chill and unmold onto a butter dish.

SUPER-NUTRITION VARIATION:

Beat in the contents of one 5,000 IU SUPER DRY A & D capsule.

VARIATION: *WHIPPED "HEALTHY BUTTER"*

Incorporating air and water increases the volume so that caloric and food values are reduced by approximately one-third for a given measure. This makes an easily spreadable table spread that may be used for seasoning but is inclined to spatter if used for sautéeing.

1 recipe Healthy Butter at room
   temperature
⅓ cup water

Prepare Healthy Butter as directed, then beat in the water with an electric mixer on high speed.

PEANUT-BUTTER BUTTER

1¼ cups NATURAL PEANUT   3 tablespoons COLD PRESSED
   BUTTER   SAFFLOWER OIL
¼ pound safflower margarine or 1 tablespoon WHEAT GERM
   butter at room temperature   OIL
                               ½ teaspoon LIQUID LECITHIN

Beat all ingredients with an electric mixer until smooth and creamy. Store in the refrigerator and use as a table spread for toast, pancakes, waffles, etc.

QUICK-FIX VARIATION: If you have "Healthy Butter" on hand, mix with peanut butter in a ratio of 2 parts peanut butter to 1 part butter.

HONEY BUTTER

¾ cup RAW HONEY   1 tablespoon COLD PRESSED
¼ pound safflower margarine or   WHEAT GERM OIL
   butter at room temperature ½ teaspoon LIQUID LECITHIN
3 tablespoons COLD PRESSED
   SAFFLOWER OIL

Beat all ingredients by hand or with an electric mixer until smooth and creamy. Store in the refrigerator in a covered container for use as a table spread. It is easily spreadable, even on unheated breads, without the bother of a dripping honey server.

HERBS & SPICES

Herbs and spices do much more than add flavor and reduce the amount of salt required for well-seasoned foods—they also add vitamins, minerals and fiber. Mild Spanish paprika, for instance, can be dusted over practically any salad, vegetable dish or entree to add visual appeal and over 1200 International Units of vitamin A per teaspoon plus appreciable amounts of potassium and fiber, half a milligram of iron, and measurable amounts of the B-complex vitamins and zinc. Even relatively small amounts of fresh herbs add fiber, iron, calcium, potassium and vitamin A.

Dried herbs and spices retain their pungency better when stored in seed or leaf form and pulverized before using. A small, inexpensive, seed or coffee mill eliminates both time and effort, but a combination of electric blender, processor, and/or a mortar and pestle will suffice.

Making your own frequently-used combinations offers multiple benefits by economizing on the original expenditures for an adequate spice collection; utilizing all of the seldom-used spices before they grow old and weak; catering to your family's preference for more sage in the poultry seasoning, less rosemary with Italian seasoning, or a milder chili powder; and avoiding the ever-present MSG in most commercial mixtures. Even though sizable amounts of supplements can be unobtrusively included with these mixtures, it seems more prudent to limit the supplements to kelp and a little vitamin C, and then add individual supplements to bolster specific dishes according to need.

CHILI POWDER

2 tablespoons crushed red pepper with seeds
1 tablespoon KELP SEASONING
1 tablespoon paprika
1 teaspoon chili pequins or tepins
1 teaspoon crushed, dried oregano
½ teaspoon garlic powder

½ teaspoon comino seed (or ¼
    teaspoon ground cumin)
½ teaspoon coriander seed (or
    ¼ teaspoon ground coriander)
¼ teaspoon C-TRATE

⅛ teaspoon ground cinnamon
2 whole allspice (or ⅛ teaspoon
    ground allspice)
1 whole clove (or pinch of ground
    cloves)

If you have whole, dried red chili peppers, wipe them
with a damp cloth, remove any stems and grind the peppers in an electric blender before measuring the 2 tablespoons.

Place all ingredients in a small electric seed mill and
process to a fine powder. Store in an air-tight spice jar.
The "heat" may be adjusted by increasing or decreasing
the amount of chili pequins used—with the one teaspoon-
ful, the chili powder is just "medium hot."

Yield: 5 tablespoons, enough to fill a small spice jar

SEASONED SALT

¼ cup SEA SALT
1 tablespoon paprika
2 teaspoons NATURAL CELERY
    SALT
2 teaspoons ARROWROOT or
    cornstarch

2 teaspoons KELP SEASONING
½ teaspoon chili powder
½ teaspoon onion powder
¼ teaspoon garlic powder
¼ teaspoon ground turmeric
⅛ teaspoon C-TRATE

Thoroughly combine all ingredients and store, tightly closed,
in a shaker-top bottle.

Yield: Approximately ½ cup

SEASONED FLOUR

1½ cups unsifted UNBLEACHED
    WHITE FLOUR
½ cup WHOLE-WHEAT
    PASTRY FLOUR
¼ cup SOY FLOUR
¼ cup non-instant SKIM MILK
    POWDER
1 teaspoon paprika

1 teaspoon KELP SEASONING
1 teaspoon SEA SALT
½ teaspoon baking powder
¼ teaspoon natural celery salt
¼ teaspoon onion powder
¼ teaspoon poultry seasoning
¼ teaspoon ground white pepper
¼ teaspoon C-TRATE

contents of 1 DAILY B-COM-
PLEX capsule (optional)   contents of 1 5,000 IU SUPER
DRY A & D capsule (optional)

Thoroughly combine all ingredients by hand with a wire whisk, with a food processor, or by beating on low speed with an electric mixer. Store in a tightly closed canister on the cupboard shelf to use for breading any type of meat, poultry or seafood. The Seasoned Flour also serves as a time-saver for making gravies and sauces.

Yield: 13 servings of 2 tablespoons each

TIME-SAVER GRAVY AND CREAM SAUCE

GRAVY: Heat 2 tablespoons of COLD PRESSED SAF-FLOWER OIL and stir in 3 tablespoons of the Seasoned Flour. Add 1 cup of chicken or beef broth and heat to boiling.

CREAM SAUCE: Heat 2 tablespoons of COLD PRESSED SAFFLOWER OIL and stir in 3 tablespoons of Seasoned Flour. Reconstitute ¼ cup SKIM MILK POWDER in 1 cup of water. Stir in and bring to boiling.

ROTISSERIE MAGIC

This mixture effectively performs its magic with cooked meat, seafood or poultry. For convenience, the dry ingredients may be mixed in quantity and stored in a tightly closed jar. Allow 1½ tablespoons for 4 servings. Mix in the sesame oil, then stir in wheat germ oil until of the desired consistency. Additional seasonings may be included to adapt to the menu: dry mustard, crushed Italian seasoning, chili powder, celery, garlic or onion salt, etc.

1½ teaspoons paprika
1 teaspoon dried parsley
½ teaspoon *each* Seasoned Salt and KELP SEASONING
¼ teaspoon B-COMPLEX POW-DER

contents of 1 5,000 IU SUPER DRY A & D capsule
⅛ teaspon *each* C-TRATE and ground white pepper
1 teaspoon *each* SESAME OIL and WHEAT GERM OIL

Mix the dry ingredients in a small dish and stir in the oils. Using a pastry brush, coat the cooked chicken, meat or seafood on all sides and heat in a conventional or microwave oven. If the food is to be served cold, see the directions for Delicatessen Chicken on page 100.

Yield: 4 servings

"INSTANT" KETCHUP

A tasty example of "making the best of both worlds"—good, old-fashioned ketchup made in fifteen minutes with modern, already-simmered tomato products and natural supplements for even better nutrition. Adding lecithin to ketchup is a wonderful way to get it "where the action is"—on meats containing saturated fats! The lecithin doesn't affect the flavor and does give the ketchup a smooth, commercial-type consistency.

½ teaspoon VEGE-SAL
¼ teaspoon dry mustard
⅛ teaspoon ground white pepper
⅔ cup water
½ cup canned tomato puree
¼ cup canned tomato paste
¼ small white onion
2 tablespoons APPLE CIDER VINEGAR

1 tablespoon BLACKSTRAP MOLASSES
2 teaspoons fresh lemon juice
¼ teaspoon Natural Liquid Smoke (optional)
¼ teaspoon C-TRATE
1 tablespoon LIQUID LECITHIN (optional)

Combine Vege-Sal, mustard and pepper in a small saucepan. Stir in water, then tomato puree and tomato paste. Using a fine grater, grate onion directly into the saucepan. Stir in with vinegar, molasses, lemon juice and smoke flavoring (if used). Cover and bring to boiling over medium heat. Stir, lower heat and simmer, uncovered, for 5 minutes.

TO MICROWAVE: Combine Vege-Sal, mustard and pepper in 4-cup glass measure. Stir in water, then tomato puree and tomato paste. Using a fine grater, grate onion directly into the tomato mixture. Stir in vinegar, molasses, lemon juice and smoke flavoring (if used). Cover with a sheet of waxed paper and microwave on full power for 5 minutes, stirring after 3 minutes.

Stir in C-Trate. (If using lecithin, pour ketchup into the container of an electric blender and blend on high speed until thoroughly combined.) Pour into a clean, hot, recycled ketchup bottle.

Yield: 1½ cups

MUSHROOM KETCHUP

This savory meat sauce is an adaptation of a table favorite from colonial times. The few seconds of whirring in an electric blender replaces days of alternately salting and pounding with a mortar and pestle, and probably retains more of the vitamins and minerals in the mushrooms.

⅓ cup "Instant" Ketchup
1 teaspoon APPLE CIDER VINEGAR
1 teaspoon BLACKSTRAP MOLASSES

1 teaspoon Worcestershire sauce
¼ pound fresh mushrooms
½ teaspoon VEGE-SAL
⅛ teaspon C-TRATE

Pour ketchup in blender container. Add vinegar, molasses and Worcestershire sauce. Rinse and dry mushrooms. Cut larger ones in half and add to blender with Vege-Sal. Blend on high speed until liquefied, pushing down sides with a rubber spatula as needed.

Pour into a small saucepan, cover and bring to boiling over medium heat. Stir, reduce heat and simmer for 5 minutes.

TO MICROWAVE: Pour into glass serving dish, cover with a paper towel and microwave on full power for 3 minutes, stirring once.

Stir C-Trate into the sauce and serve with meatloaf, roasts or steaks.

Mushroom Ketchup will keep in the refrigerator for several weeks and makes a savory addition to cold meats or sandwiches.

Yield: ¾ cup

QUICK & EASY TOMATO SAUCE

The tomato paste and chicken broth have had their long simmering—so the few minutes of cooking produces a full-bodied sauce that is both economical and nutritious. For added convenience, double the recipe (increasing microwave cooking times by one-third) and freeze the sauce in one-cup containers. Adding various seasonings just before serving individualizes the sauce— basil for Italian dishes, cumin and additional chili powder for Mexican, etc; or experiment with the variations listed.

2 tablespoons minced onion
2 tablespoons minced green bell pepper
1 teaspoon COLD PRESSED ALL BLEND OIL
1 tablespoon SOY FLOUR
½ teaspoon seasoned salt
½ teaspoon KELP SEASONING
½ teaspoon paprika
¼ teaspoon chili powder

1 cup canned tomato paste
1 cup chicken broth, homemade or canned
1 cup water
2 teaspoons BLACKSTRAP MOLASSES
1 tablespoon LIQUID LECITHIN
¼ teaspoon C-TRATE

Sauté onion and pepper in the oil until limp. Sprinkle on flour and stir in with salt, kelp, paprika and chili powder. Stir in tomato paste, broth, water and molasses. Bring to a boil, lower heat and simmer, uncovered, for 10 minutes. Whisk in lecithin and C-Trate.

TO MICROWAVE: Combine onion, pepper and oil in a 1½ or 2-quart casserole and microwave on full power for 3 minutes, uncovered. Stir in soy flour, salt, kelp, paprika and chili powder. Blend in tomato paste, broth, ¾ cup water and molasses. Microwave on full power, uncovered, until mixture is fully boiling—about 5 minutes. Whisk in lecithin and vitamin C powder.

Yield: 2½ cups

VARIATION #1—*FRESH TOMATO SAUCE*

⅔ cup Quick & Easy Tomato Sauce
1 teaspoon BREWER'S YEAST

¼ teaspoon natural celery salt
¼ teaspoon KELP SEASONING
1 ripe salad tomato

Whisk brewer's yeast, celery salt and kelp seasoning into the sauce. Wash, core and finely chop the tomato. Stir into the sauce. (Or blend the sauce with the dry ingredients in an electric blender. Wash and core the tomato. Cut in quarters and blend until finely chopped.) Heat the sauce to serving temperature on the stove or in the microwave oven.

Yield: 1 cup

VARIATION #2—*MUSHROOM-TOMATO SAUCE*

⅔ cup Quick & Easy Tomato Sauce
1 teaspoon BREWER'S YEAST
¼ teaspoon onion powder
¼ teaspoon KELP SEASONING
⅛ teaspoon SEA SALT

⅛ teaspoon crushed, dried marjoram
¼ cup chopped, drained canned mushrooms plus 1 tablespoon of liquid

Combine all ingredients except mushrooms with a wire whisk or in an electric blender. Stir in mushrooms (or add to blender and whir for a few seconds). Heat to serving temperature on the stove or in the microwave oven.

Yield: 1 cup

⅔ cup Quick & Easy Tomato Sauce

½ cup shredded (2 ounces) sharp
natural cheddar cheese

2 teaspoons BREWER'S YEAST

½ teaspoon RAW BROWN
SUGAR

½ teaspoon chili powder

¼ teaspoon SEA SALT

1 ripe salad tomato

2 tablespoons chopped, canned
green chilies with seeds

Combine all ingredients except tomato and green chiles.
Wash and core tomato and chop very fine. Stir in with
green chiles.

> **WITH ELECTRIC BLENDER:** Measure sauce in
> blender container. Cut cheese in half-inch cubes and
> blend on medium speed with yeast, brown sugar, chili
> powder and salt. Wash, core and quarter tomato.
> Add to blender with green chiles and blend until
> tomato is finely chopped.

Heat to serving temperature on the stove or in a microwave oven.

Yield: 1½ cups

SLOW & EASY TOMATO SAUCE

_This long-simmered, all-purpose sauce becomes extra nourishing
and delicious when the chopped meat melts into the liquid, but
either version has a chameleon-like quality of adapting to the
cuisine of the day. Use it for any of the Quick Tomato Sauce
variations or stir in some chopped basil and serve it over hot,
cooked pasta with sprinklings of grated Parmesan cheese. For a
complete change of nationality, mix 1 cup of the sauce with 1
tablespoon Tamari Soy Sauce blended with 1 teaspoon ARROW-
ROOT; then heat and serve as a dipping sauce for seafood or
won-ton._

1 tablespoon COLD PRESSED
VIRGIN OLIVE OIL

1 large rib celery, with leaves,
chopped

½ medium onion, chopped

½ large green bell pepper,
chopped with core and seeds

4 cups canned tomatoes and liquid (2 16-ounce cans)

1 large carrot

1 garlic clove
1 cup (8 ounces) lean, trimmed round steak or beef roast, in ¼-inch dice (optional)
1 4-ounce can mushroom stems and pieces with liquid (optional)
1 6-ounce can tomato paste
2 cups beef broth, homemade or canned
¼ cup snipped fresh parsley or 2 tablespoons dried parsley
2 tablespoons BLACKSTRAP MOLASSES
2 teaspoons SEA SALT
1½ teaspoons paprika
1 teaspoon KELP SEASONING
½ teaspoon crushed, dried Italian seasoning
¼ teaspoon ground black pepper

Sauté celery, onion and bell pepper in olive oil until limp. Spoon into the container of an electric blender and puree with 1 cup of the canned tomatoes. Pour into a 3½ to 4 quart slow-cooker or a large saucepan for range-top cooking. Cut carrot into 1-inch sections and puree in the blender with the garlic and remaining tomatoes. (Or break up the tomatoes and stir into the slow-cooker or saucepan with hand-grated carrots.) Stir in with beef and mushrooms (if used) and remaining ingredients. Cover and cook over low heat on the range top for 6 to 8 hours, stirring occasionally; or set on Low in the covered slow-cooker and let simmer for 12 to 18 hours. Thicken sauce, if desired, by slightly increasing the heat and cooking without a cover for the last hour, or by blending in 1 tablespoon of arrowroot mixed with 1 tablespoon water.

Any sauce not used immediately may be frozen in small containers, then popped out for freezer storage in a plastic bag.

Yield: 7 cups meatless sauce
8 cups meat and mushroom sauce

ALMOST SOUR CREAM & CHIVES

Higher in nourishment and lower in calories than either sour cream or the "plastic" potato toppings, this rich-tasting blend offers salvation for weight watchers as well as the health and/or economy conscious.

1 cup low-fat cottage cheese (recipe for homemade on page 51)
3 tablespoons ACIDOPHILUS
   YOGURT

2 tablespoons grated Parmesan
   cheese
¼ teaspoon C-TRATE
Crisp tops from 3 green onions
   (3 tablespoons, minced)

Sieve cottage cheese into a mixing bowl and blend with yogurt, Parmesan cheese and C-Trate until smooth. Mince onion tops and stir in.

> **WITH FOOD PROCESSOR:** In work bowl with cutting blade, place cottage cheese, yogurt, Parmesan cheese and C-Trate. Process until smooth. Cut onion tops into half-inch sections and drop through the feed tube with the processor running normally.

Refrigerate in a covered serving dish. (Mixture thickens when chilled and may be thinned with additional yogurt or skim milk, if desired.)

Yield: 1¼ cup

CURRIED PEACHES & PEARS

Add the excitement of an Indian curry to plain poultry, meats, or sandwiches with this easily prepared relish—and add some needed nutrients as well. It improves with age as the flavors mellow, so the amounts can be doubled and the curry stored in the refrigerator in a covered container.

1 tablespoon safflower margarine
1 tablespoon RAW HONEY
1 teaspoon curry powder

¼ teaspoon SEA SALT
1 large peach (6 ounces)
1 large pear (6 ounces)

Melt margarine in a small baking dish and blend in honey. Mix curry powder with salt and stir in. Peel peach, remove pit and quarter, then cut in ¼-inch crosswise slices. Quarter pear, remove core but peel only if the skin is tough. Cut in short, ¼-inch slices and stir into the curry mixture with the peach. Cover and bake in a preheated 350 degree oven for 30 minutes.

TO MICROWAVE: Melt margarine in a glass jar or serving dish by microwaving on full power for 1 minute. Blend in honey. Mix curry powder with salt and stir in. Prepare fruit as directed and stir in. Cover and microwave on full power for 5 minutes, stirring once.

SUPER-NUTRITION VARIATION:

● Add with the salt: ¼ teaspoon additional curry powder
¼ teaspoon B-COMPLEX POWDER
⅛ teaspoon C-TRATE
contents of 1 5,000 IU SUPER DRY A & D capsule

● Add ¼ cup RAISINS with the peaches and pears

Yield: 6 servings

NUTTY NECTARINE SAUCE

A fresh fruit sauce that can be prepared in advance, frozen, then defrosted and warmed to serve over molded puddings, ice cream, gingerbread, plain cake, waffles, or ice-cream-filled crepes.

1 cup finely chopped fresh nectarines	3 tablespoons ARROWROOT or cornstarch
¼ teaspoon C-TRATE	⅛ teaspoon ground cloves
⅓ cup chopped walnuts	⅛ teaspoon SEA SALT
1 tablespoon safflower margarine, cut in quarters	¾ cup orange juice
⅓ cup RAW BROWN SUGAR	¼ cup ORANGE BLOSSOM HONEY

Wash and pit nectarines; remove blemishes but do not peel. Cut into ¼-inch cubes and toss with C-Trate. Set aside.

In a small pan, cook and stir nuts and margarine until bubbling—about 4 minutes. Set aside.

In a quart saucepan, combine brown sugar, arrowroot,

cloves and salt. Blend in orange juice and honey. Cook
and stir over medium-low heat until thickened and clear—
about 10 minutes. Stir in nut and nectarine mixtures.

TO MICROWAVE: Prepare nectarines, toss with C-
Trate and set aside. Combine nuts with margarine in
a small dish and microwave, uncovered, for 2 minutes on full power. Set aside. In a 4-cup measure,
combine brown sugar, arrowroot, cloves and salt.
Blend in orange juice and honey. Microwave 4 minutes on full power, stirring once each minute. Stir in
nut and nectarine mixtures.

If sauce is thicker than desired, thin with water or orange
juice before serving.

VARIATION: *GINGER PEACHY SAUCE*

Substitute: Peeled chopped fresh peaches for nectarines
             Pecans for walnuts
             ½ teaspoon ground ginger for the ⅛ teaspoon
             ground cloves

Yield: 1 pint

FIG DESSERT SAUCE

*This flavor combination offers total concealment for the yogurt
and an opportunity for everyone to reap a few of its benefits.*

½ cup ACIDOPHILUS YO-
GURT

½ cup RAW HONEY

2 tablespoons non-instant SKIM
MILK POWDER

1 cup chopped fresh Black Mission Figs or ½ cup chopped
dried figs

¼ teaspoon C-TRATE

Blend yogurt, honey and skim milk powder in an electric
blender. Add figs and C-Trate and blend until smooth.

Serve over plain cake, ice cream or frozen yogurt.

Yield: 1⅓ cups = 6 servings

VARIATION: *MISSION SHERBET*

Make sauce as directed, then blend in ½ cup orange juice.
Freeze until slushy and serve as a fruited sherbet.

Yield: 4 servings

ALMOST MAPLE SYRUP

*For the times when honey or a fruit syrup won't quite fill the bill,
try this maple syrup with old-fashioned flavor but only half the
calories and carbohydrates of commercial brands.*

½ cup FRUCTOSE GRANULES
½ cup RAW BROWN SUGAR
1 tablespoon ARROWROOT or
  cornstarch
¹⁄₁₆ teaspoon SEA SALT

1 cup warm water
1 teaspoon BLACKSTRAP
  MOLASSES
¼ teaspoon pure maple flavoring

Combine fructose, brown sugar, arrowroot and salt in a
small saucepan. Stir in water and molasses. Cook and stir
over low heat until boiling. Remove from heat and stir in
flavoring.

TO MICROWAVE: Combine fructose, brown sugar,
arrowroot and salt with water and molasses in a 4-cup
glass measure. Microwave 3 minutes—or until fully
boiling. Stir in flavoring.

Any syrup not used immediately may be refrigerated in
a glass bottle. Warm before serving by removing bottle
cap and heating in a pan of hot water or in the microwave
oven for a few seconds. Stir or re-cap and shake before
serving.

Yield: 1¾ cups

COMPARISON CHART

	Corn Syrup*	Pure Maple Syrup*	Almost Maple Syrup
per 1 tablespoon			
Calories	57	50	28
Carbohydrates, grams	14.8	12.8	7.7
Iron, milligrams	.8	.2	.2
Potassium, milligrams	1.	26.	21.

*from USDA *Bulletin #72* and *Nutrition Almanac*, McGraw Hill Paperback, New York, 1979.

CHAPTER 7

BREADS

CREPES
PANCAKES & WAFFLES
MUFFINS & CORNBREAD
LOAF BREADS & ROLLS

CREPES

Crepes are a lovely example of cooking as a creative art: using the same ingredients you can serve a mundane supper of hash, eggs, bread and milk; or an elegant French repast of filled crepes with a bubbling sauce. The crepes themselves offer interesting ways to incorporate whole grains in the menu, and the fillings are golden opportunities for fortifying leftovers with all sorts of supplemental nourishment. Preparation and storage are so easy that crepes rate as "emergency rations" for the cook. Filled or unfilled, crepes may be covered and refrigerated for a day or so, or frozen for weeks and quickly thawed for impromptu meals or snacks.

BASIC CREPES

1 cup STONE-GROUND WHOLE WHEAT FLOUR	1½ cups water
⅓ cup non-instant SKIM MILK POWDER	4 large eggs
	1 tablespoon LIQUID LECITHIN
¼ teaspoon SEA SALT	1 teaspoon SAFFLOWER OIL

Combine flour, skim milk powder and salt in a mixing bowl. Blend in the water, then whisk in the eggs, lecithin and oil—or beat with a rotary beater. (This batter is now ready for making crepes—if an electric mixer, blender or food processor is used, air is incorporated and the batter should stand for an hour before using.)

Cook crepes according to the instructions with your crepe pan or heat a small, lightly greased skillet. Lift it from the heat and pour in 2 tablespoons of batter, tilting the skillet to spread the batter to make a thin, six-inch pancake. Cook until golden brown on one side only and slide onto a paper towel. Repeat with remainder of the batter, stacking the crepes with layers of waxed paper.

VARIATIONS:

- Add 2 tablespoons of RICE BRAN, SOY FLOUR or WHEAT GERM to the batter

- Substitute ¼ cup BARLEY FLOUR, OATMEAL FLOUR, MILLET FLOUR or RYE FLOUR for ¼ cup of the whole wheat flour

- For crepes to wrap around Spanish or Mexican fillings, substitute ⅓ cup YELLOW CORNMEAL for ⅓ cup of the whole wheat flour

- For sensational Graham Cracker Dessert Crepes: substitute GRAHAM FLOUR for the whole wheat and beat in 2 teaspoons of RAW HONEY with the liquid lecithin.

Note: Bran, wheat germ and many of the whole-grain flours are inclined to settle to the bottom of the batter and should be stirred occasionally while making the crepes.

Yield: 18 thin crepes

SPINACH-PEPITA CREPES

Pumpkin Seed Meal (ground pepitas) not only tastes exotically delicious and furnishes calcium, phosphorus, iron, fiber, B vitamins and zinc, but also acts as a binder for the filling. Either the chicken or cheese crepes may be prepared ahead of time and frozen for impressive meals on short notice.

CHICKEN-SPINACH PEPITA CREPES

FILLING:

1 tablespoon safflower margarine

2 thinly sliced green onions with crisp tops

¼ pound fresh mushrooms, sliced

½ 10-ounce package frozen, chopped spinach

½ cup (2 ounces) finely chopped or shredded Monterey Jack cheese

¼ cup PUMPKIN SEED MEAL

2 tablespoons ACIDOPHILUS	1 tablespoon apple juice or
YOGURT	Marsala wine
1 cup diced cooked chicken	½ teaspoon SPIKE

Melt margarine in skillet and sauté onion with sliced mushrooms until onion is limp but not browned. Cook spinach according to package directions and drain, pressing with a spoon to remove excess moisture. Stir into the onion mixture with cheese, pumpkin seed meal and yogurt, then stir in chicken, apple juice and Spike. Set aside.

TO MICROWAVE: Place frozen spinach in a 1-quart cooking dish, cover and microwave for 5 minutes on full power, stirring after 3 minutes. Transfer to a sieve to drain. Wipe dish with a paper towel and microwave the margarine for 30 seconds on full power. Stir in onions and mushrooms. Microwave on full power, uncovered, for 3 minutes—stirring after 2 minutes. Stir in drained spinach and all other ingredients. Set aside.

SWISS CREAM SAUCE

1 tablespoon COLD PRESSED	3 tablespoons non-instant SKIM
SAFFLOWER OIL	MILK POWDER
1 tablespoon safflower	1 tablespoon SOY FLOUR
margarine	1 teaspoon BREWER'S YEAST
2 tablespoons UNBLEACHED	¼ teaspoon SEA SALT
WHITE FLOUR	¼ cup shredded natural Swiss
1 cup chicken broth, homemade	cheese (1 ounce)
or canned	

Melt margarine with oil in a small saucepan. Stir in white flour and cook and stir until bubbly. Measure broth in blender container and add dry milk, soy flour and brewer's yeast. Blend until smooth (or whisk in a small bowl). Stir into the flour mixture with cheese and salt. Cook and stir until the sauce thickens and boils.

TO MICROWAVE: Microwave oil and margarine in a 2-cup glass measure for 30 seconds. Stir in white flour and microwave for 1 minute. Place broth, skim milk powder, soy flour and brewer's yeast in the container of an electric blender and whir until smooth (or whisk together in a small bowl). Stir into flour and microwave 4 minutes on full power, stirring twice—sauce should be thickened and boiling. Stir in salt and cheese and let stand to melt.

To assemble crepes: Spread 3 tablespoons of the filling in a strip down the center of each crepe. Fold in each side to overlap the filling and place, folded-side up, in a shallow baking dish. Pour sauce over the crepes, leaving the ends exposed. Bake in a preheated 350 degree oven for 15 minutes or microwave for 5 minutes on full power, rotating the dish after 3 minutes. (For even microwave heating, arrange the filled crepes in an extra large baking dish so that a blank space can be left in the center, then elevate the dish on a rack or an inverted baking dish so the microwaves can penetrate from the under side.)

Yield: fills 8 Basic Crepes

SUBSTITUTIONS: Crepes encourage flexibility in recipes and all manner of substitutions may be made in this one without affecting the flavor or appreciably altering the nutritional analysis.

● A drained, 2-ounce can of sliced mushrooms will take the place of the fresh mushrooms

● ½ cup leftover, cooked, drained, chopped spinach may be used in place of the frozen chopped spinach

● Swiss cheese will substitute for Monterey Jack cheese

● Sour cream can replace the yogurt

● Cornmeal or any other variation of the Basic Crepes can be used

● Mushroom or any cream sauce will substitute for the Swiss Cream Sauce

VEGETARIAN VARIATION: *CHEESE-SPINACH PEPITA CREPES*

Omit mushrooms, chicken and apple juice from the Chicken-Spinach filling

Add: 1 cup low fat cottage cheese, sieved or pureed in the processor

2 tablespoons grated Parmesan cheese

⅛ teaspoon *each* ground black pepper and ground mace

Prepare as for the chicken filling, thoroughly blending all ingredients. Place 3 tablespoons of filling off center on a crepe, approximately 1½ inches from one end and leaving a 1½-inch margin on each side. Fold the end over the filling and fold in both sides, then roll up to make a spill-proof cylinder about 4 inches long and 1 inch in diameter. Repeat with remaining crepes and filling. Arrange rolls, seam-side down in an oiled baking dish and pour sauce (prepared with water instead of chicken broth) over the tops. Bake in a preheated, 350 degree oven for 15 minutes; or microwave, uncovered, for 5 minutes on full power, rotating the dish after 3 minutes.

SUPER-NUTRITION VARIATION FOR EITHER CHICKEN OR CHEESE FILLING:

● Stir into the filling with the seasonings:

2 tablespoons LECITHIN GRANULES

1 teaspoon GRANULATED KELP contents of 1 DAILY B capsule

⅛ teaspoon C-TRATE

Yield: 4 servings of 2 crepes each

PLANNED-OVER CREPES

Small amounts of leftovers (planned-overs sound decidedly more enticing) become exciting entrees when folded in a crepe and topped with whatever sauce or gravy has been hibernating in the refrigerator. These Broccoli Cheese Crepes offer an excellent

pattern that can be adapted to whatever meats or vegetables are available, can be doubled in quantity to serve four, and/or can have the super-nutrition supplements added. (No food composition figures are given because of the variables.)

BROCCOLI-CHEESE CREPES FOR TWO

1 teaspoon SAFFLOWER OIL
2 tablespoons sliced green
   onions with crisp tops
2 tablespoons chopped, drained,
   canned mushrooms
½ cup chopped cooked chicken
½ cup chopped cooked broccoli

¼ cup (1 ounce) shredded or
   finely chopped Monterey Jack
   cheese
1 tablespoon LECITHIN
   GRANULES
½ teaspoon KELP
   SEASONING
4 Basic Crepes

Stir onions into the oil in a small skillet and sauté until limp. Stir in remaining ingredients and spoon one-fourth of the filling down the centers of each crepe. Fold in one-third of the crepe on each side and place in a baking dish with the folded sides up. Spoon 2 tablespoons of any cream sauce atop each crepe and heat to serving temperature in a conventional or microwave oven.

SAMPLE VARIATIONS:

● Substitute chopped or shredded cooked beef for the chicken and use sharp natural cheddar cheese in place of the Monterey Jack cheese. Top crepes with beef gravy, tomato sauce or any cream sauce.

● Substitute flaked, cooked fish for the chicken, sliced green grapes for the mushrooms, and use either Monterey Jack or Swiss cheese. Stir a spoonful of white wine or apple juice into the cream sauce before spooning over the filled crepes.

OLD-FASHIONED BUCKWHEAT PANCAKES

"Making a sponge" was the old-fashioned method of coping with the earlier forms of yeast. For us it is a morning time-saver. By preparing the batter the night before, real pancakes for breakfast are possible, even on working days. These cakes have genuine

buckwheat flavor and goodness, plus a little something extra from the bran, honey and skim milk powder. Serve with Almost Maple Syrup (recipe on page 165) for a special treat and an especially good start for the day.

1¼ cups water	1 tablespoon COLD
1 tablespoon RAW	PRESSED ALL BLEND OIL
HONEY	½ cup non-instant SKIM MILK
1 teaspoon ACTIVE DRY	POWDER
YEAST	¼ cup unprocessed PURE
¾ cup unsifted	BRAN
UNBLEACHED WHITE	½ teaspoon SEA SALT
FLOUR	1 large egg
½ cup BUCKWHEAT	
FLOUR	

The night before you will want pancakes for breakfast: Heat water and honey to 115 degrees and pour over yeast in a large mixing bowl. Let stand 5 minutes, or until foamy. Add white flour, buckwheat flour and oil. Beat 3 minutes on medium speed with an electric mixer or 50 strokes by hand. Beat in skim milk powder, bran and salt. Cover and let stand for 8 to 12 hours at room temperature.

When ready to serve: Beat the egg into the batter and bake on a hot griddle until golden brown.

SUPER-NUTRITION VARIATION:

• Use ¾ cup STONE-GROUND WHOLE WHEAT FLOUR in place of the unbleached white flour

• When beating in the egg, add:
   3 tablespoons LECITHIN GRANULES
   1 tablespoon BREWER'S YEAST
   ½ teaspoon DOLOMITE POWDER

Yield: Twelve 4-inch pancakes

YEAST WAFFLES

To paraphrase the bakery goods commercial, "Nobody doesn't like waffles," so the glamorous crepe makers shouldn't be al-

lowed to relegate the waffle iron to a dark corner of the cupboard. Waffles are equally versatile and can serve as a short-cake base for luncheon or dinner entrees or desserts as well as the traditional "special" for breakfast. The waffles may be made in quantity and frozen for instant defrosting in a microwave or toaster oven, and can camouflage a lot of health-giving nutrients in each delicious bite. Using yeast as the leavening agent prevents any possible loss of B vitamins or calcium, requires only an extra 15 minutes of rising time when mixing the batter, and produces blissfully light and delicate waffles.

BASIC WAFFLES

An all-purpose waffle for serving with syrup at breakfast; topped with creamed beef, chicken or seafood as a main dish; or layered with fruit and whipped topping for dessert.

2 tablespoons RAW HONEY
1¾ cups warm water (115 degrees) divided
1 tablespoon active dry yeast
¾ cup WHOLE WHEAT PASTRY FLOUR
¾ cup unsifted UNBLEACHED WHITE FLOUR
½ cup non-instant SKIM MILK POWDER
¼ cup toasted WHEAT GERM
1 tablespoon BREWER'S YEAST
½ teaspoon SEA SALT
2 tablespoons COLD PRESSED ALL BLEND OIL
1 tablespoon LIQUID LECITHIN
2 large eggs, separated
¼ cup LECITHIN GRANULES

WITH ELECTRIC MIXER OR ROTARY BEATER:
Stir honey into ½ cup of the warm water in a large mixing bowl. Sprinkle yeast on the surface and let stand for 5 minutes, or until foamy.

In a small mixing bowl, combine the flours, skim milk powder, wheat germ, brewer's yeast and salt. Add to the yeast mixture with the remaining water, oil, liquid lecithin and egg yolks. Beat on low speed for 2 minutes, or by hand for 40 strokes. Cover and let stand for 15 minutes.

Beat egg whites in the small mixing bowl until stiff but not dry. Fold into the batter with the lecithin granules. Bake in a waffle iron according to the manufacturer's directions.

WITH FOOD PROCESSOR: Sprinkle yeast on ½ cup of the warm water in a small dish and let stand for 5 minutes, or until foamy.

In processor bowl with mixing blade, place flours, skim milk powder, wheat germ, brewer's yeast and salt. Blend with 3 pulsations or on/off turns.

Add yeast mixture, oil, liquid lecithin, honey and egg yolks. With processor running normally, add the remaining 1¼ cups of water through the feed tube. Let stand 15 minutes for the yeast to develop.

Beat egg whites until stiff but not dry. Fold in the batter and the lecithin granules. Bake in a waffle iron according to the manufacturer's directions.

VARIATIONS:

● Add 2 tablespoons SOY FLOUR, PURE BRAN or RICE BRAN with the wheat and white flours

● Substitute ¼ cup BUCKWHEAT FLOUR, MILLET FLOUR, OAT FLOUR or RICE FLOUR for ¼ cup of the unbleached white flour

Yield: Ten 6-inch round waffles

OATMEAL ENTREE WAFFLES

Topped with Salmon Newburg (recipe on page 109) and accompanied by steamed broccoli and fresh tomato slices, these savory waffles make a heartily satisfying meal that is strikingly attractive and chock full of vitamins and minerals with the protein equiva-

lent of two eggs in each waffle. (Meal totals are included in the Nutritional Analysis Tables following the Salmon Newburg entry.)

¾ cup warm chicken broth (115 degrees)
1½ teaspoons active dry yeast
⅔ cup ROLLED OATS
⅓ cup STONE-GROUND WHOLE WHEAT FLOUR
⅓ cup non-instant SKIM MILK POWDER

1 tablespoon BREWER'S YEAST
½ teaspoon SPIKE
1 large egg, separated
1 egg white
2 tablespoons LIQUID LECITHIN

Sprinkle yeast on warm broth in a mixing bowl. Let stand for 5 minutes, or until foamy. Combine oats, flour, skim milk powder, brewer's yeast and Spike. Stir into yeast mixture with egg yolk and lecithin. Beat for 3 minutes with an electric mixer or 50 strokes by hand. Let stand 15 minutes.

WITH ELECTRIC BLENDER: Sprinkle yeast on the chicken broth in a small bowl and let stand for 5 minutes, or until foamy. Grind oats for 10 seconds in the blender. Add flour, skim milk powder, brewer's yeast and Spike. Blend on low speed for 10 seconds, then invert the covered container to loosen the material under the blades. Replace the container, add yeast mixture, egg yolk and lecithin. Blend on medium speed until smooth, scraping down sides with a rubber spatula as needed. Let stand for 15 minutes.

Beat egg whites until stiff but not dry. Fold in the batter and bake in a waffle iron according to the manufacturer's directions.

VARIATION: Substitute beef broth for chicken broth if the waffles are to be served with beef or pork mixtures.

Yield: 4 round waffles = 4 servings

CORN WAFFLES

The high-protein ingredients neutralize the excess acid from the yogurt so no vitamin-destroying soda need be used in these flavorful breakfast or entree waffles.

¼ cup warm water (115 degrees)
1½ teaspoons active dry yeast
½ cup STONE-GROUND WHOLE WHEAT FLOUR
¼ cup non-instant SKIM MILK POWDER
¼ cup WHOLE-GROUND YELLOW CORNMEAL
2 tablespoons GLUTEN FLOUR
1 teaspoon SPIKE

2 tablespoons COLD PRESSED ALL BLEND OIL
1 tablespoon LIQUID LECITHIN
½ cup ACIDOPHILUS YOGURT
1 large egg, separated
1 egg white
¾ cup cream corn
¼ cup LECITHIN GRANULES

Sprinkle yeast on warm water in a large mixing bowl. Let stand for 5 minutes, or until foamy. In a 2-cup measure, mix wheat flour, dry milk, cornmeal, gluten flour and Spike. Add half the mixture to the yeast and water. Stir in oil, liquid lecithin, yogurt and egg yolk. Beat for 2 minutes with an electric mixer on medium speed or 40 strokes by hand. Stir in the rest of the blended dry ingredients, cover and let stand for 15 minutes.

Stir corn and lecithin granules into the batter. Beat egg whites until stiff but not dry and fold in. Bake according to directions with your waffle iron. Serve topped with barbecued meat in sauce, chili con carne, or creamed poultry, beef or seafood.

VARIATIONS:

- Substitute sour cream for the yogurt
- Alfalfa sprout Corn Waffles: Add 1 cup chopped ALFALFA SPROUTS with the corn
- Breakfast Corn Waffles: Substitute ½ teaspoon SEA SALT for the SPIKE
- Add 1 tablespoon RAW HONEY with the yogurt

SUPER-NUTRITION VARIATION: Add any or all of the following supplements as needed to balance the menu:

- 1 tablespoon BREWER'S YEAST, ¼ teaspoon B-COMPLEX POWDER and/or the contents of 1 5,000 or 10,000 IU SUPER DRY A & D capsule stirred into the dry ingredients.
- 2 additional tablespoons of LECITHIN GRANULES stirred in with the corn

Yield: six 6-inch round waffles = 6 servings

SUGAR-HONEY GRAHAM WAFFLES
(for breakfast or dessert)

1 cup warm water (115 degrees)	½ teaspoon SEA SALT
2 tablespoons RAW BROWN SUGAR	¼ cup safflower margarine, at room temperature
1½ teaspoons active dry yeast	3 tablespoons RAW HONEY
1 cup GRAHAM FLOUR	2 tablespoons LIQUID LECITHIN
½ cup non-instant SKIM MILK POWDER	2 large eggs, separated
¼ cup toasted WHEAT GERM	1 large egg white
1 tablespoon BREWER's YEAST	½ teaspoon pure vanilla

Stir sugar into water in large mixing bowl and sprinkle yeast on the surface. Let stand for 5 minutes, or until foamy.

In a 2-cup measure, combine graham flour, dry milk, wheat germ, brewer's yeast and salt. Stir into yeast mixture with margarine, honey, liquid lecithin and egg yolks. Beat for 2 minutes on medium speed with an electric mixer or 40 strokes by hand. Beat egg whites until stiff and fold into the batter with the vanilla. Bake in a waffle iron according to the manufacturer's directions.

Serve with syrup, Peanut-Butter Butter (page 152) and jelly or Honey-Butter (page 152) for breakfast. As a dinner dessert, spoon on a fruit sauce (pages 163-164) and top with a dollop of whipped topping.

Yield: Six 6-inch waffles = 6 servings

180

POCKET BREADS

Also known as pita, Syrian or Arab Bread, these round, flat breads with a natural pocket are so wonderfully convenient for sandwiches that they are gaining popularity throughout America. Surprisingly, these delightful breads are very easy to make, with each round of dough obligingly puffing into a perfect pocket with only a few minutes of baking in a conventional oven. In addition to being marvelous containers for all manner of nutritious fillings, they offer an opportunity for incorporating more whole-grain goodness into quick meals—and can change their nationality when you include cornmeal or rye flour. Homemade pocket breads also can vary in size from three-inch appetizers to eight-inch spectaculars for Dagwood-style sandwiches. For everyday practicality, reducing the standard six-inch bakery size to five inches has several advantages: all six of them can be baked at once on one large cookie sheet, one five-inch pocket bread satisfies average appetites, and they fit nicely into plastic sandwich bags for the lunchbox brigade.

BASIC WHEAT POCKETS

¾ cup warm water (115 degrees)
1 teaspoon RAW HONEY
1 tablespoon active dry yeast
1 tablespoon LIQUID LECITHIN

¾ cup unsifted, UNBLEACHED WHITE FLOUR
1 cup STONE-GROUND WHOLE WHEAT FLOUR
1 tablespoon toasted WHEAT GERM
¾ teaspoon SEA SALT

Stir honey into warm water in a mixing bowl and let stand 5 minutes, or until foamy. Add liquid lecithin and white flour. Beat for 2 minutes with an electric mixer or 60 strokes by hand. Stir in wheat flour, wheat germ and salt, kneading in the last of the flour by hand, if necessary.

WITH A FOOD PROCESSOR: Combine water and honey in processor bowl with mixing blade. Sprinkle yeast on the surface and let stand for 5 minutes, or until foamy. Add lecithin and white flour. Process for 1 minute. Add whole-wheat flour, wheat germ and salt. Process until dough gathers into a ball—about 10 seconds. Turn the dough out of the processor onto a floured surface and knead a few times to make a compact roll.

Divide dough into 6 small balls and roll each one to a 5-inch circle on a floured surface. (Roll from the center of the ball toward the outside, using as few strokes as possible—over-rolling can inhibit the puffing.) Place the rounds on a greased cookie sheet, cover with waxed paper and/or a dish towel and let rise until almost double in thickness—about 20 minutes.

To Bake Pocket Breads with a Top Broiler: Preheat oven to 475 degrees. Place the cookie sheet with the breads on the lowest oven shelf and bake for 3 or 4 minutes— bottoms should not get brown. Turn oven off and turn on top broiler. Move the cookie sheet to the highest shelf and leave until the tops are golden—about 2 minutes.

To Bake Pocket Breads without a Top Broiler: Preheat oven to 450 degrees. Place the cookie sheet with the breads on a shelf in the center of the oven and bake approximately 10 minutes.

NOTE #1: Overbaking is a temptation that should be resisted—it creates tough breads.

NOTE #2: If you make pocket breads on a rotten day and some of them refuse to puff, simply slit them with a knife before serving.

SUPER-NUTRITION VARIATION:

- Add ¼ teaspoon DOLOMITE POWDER and the contents of 1 DAILY B-COMPLEX capsule with the salt.

Yield: 6 pocket breads

ALL-STAR 95% PROTEIN SUPREME POCKET BREADS

Ideal for hypoglycemics and carbohydrate counters, each pocket bread contains 10.9 grams of protein and 24.5 grams of carbohydrate. (To compare with standard whole wheat bread: An equal amount, 63 grams, contains 5.7 grams of protein and 31 grams of carbohydrate.) No complete nutritional analysis is possible in foods made with gluten flour as the amounts of the B vitamins, iron and magnesium have not been determined.

- Omit honey
- Substitute ¼ cup GLUTEN FLOUR for ¼ cup of the unbleached white flour before beating or processing
- Substitute 1 ounce ALL-STAR 95% PROTEIN SUPREME POWDER for ¼ cup of the whole wheat flour

GLUTEN POCKET BREADS

Each of these pocket breads contains 7.3 grams of protein and 29.3 grams of carbohydrate.

- Substitute ¼ cup GLUTEN FLOUR for ¼ cup of the unbleached white flour before beating or processing.

VARIATION: *CORNMEAL POCKET BREADS*

For fiesta fare, fill with any favorite taco or enchilada filling, or mashed pinto beans, and top with shredded lettuce and cheese, chopped tomatoes and onions, plus a dash of fiery hot sauce or salsa.

- Add 2 tablespoons GLUTEN FLOUR with the unbleached white flour
- Substitute ½ cup YELLOW CORNMEAL for ½ cup of the whole wheat flour
- Omit wheat germ

VARIATION: *RYE POCKET BREADS*

These make glorious Reuben sandwiches with layers of home-corned beef, sliced turkey, Swiss cheese and drained sauerkraut . . . or great turkey-ham and cheese sandwiches with a dollop of mustard and a handful of alfalfa sprouts.

- Substitute 1 teaspoon BLACKSTRAP MOLASSES for the honey
- Substitute 100% NATURAL RYE FLOUR for the whole wheat flour
- Add ½ teaspoon ground caraway seed with the salt

ELECTRIC-MIXER POCKET BREADS

Once you and your family become addicted to pocket breads, you may want to increase the quantity and use an electric mixer for the beating.

1½ cups 115 degree water
2 teaspoons RAW HONEY
2 tablespoons active dry yeast
2 tablespoons LIQUID LECITHIN
1½ cups unsifted, UNBLEACHED WHITE FLOUR

2 cups STONE-GROUND, WHOLE WHEAT FLOUR
2 tablespoons toasted WHEAT GERM
1½ teaspoons SEA SALT

Combine water and honey in a large mixer bowl and sprinkle yeast on the surface. Let stand for 5 minutes, or until foamy.

Add lecithin and white flour. Beat on medium speed for 4 or 5 minutes. (The exact length of beating time is determined by the dough: it will start to climb the beaters when it has had enough.) Stir in remaining ingredients, turn out on a floured surface and shape into twelve 5-inch or 24 appetizer rounds. Let rise and bake as for Basic Pockets.

REGULATION MUFFINS

A delicious, natural answer to the television-commercial question, "Are you troubled by irregularity?" These light and tender muffins not only taste great but provide nutrients not offered by whatever the commercial had to sell.

½ cup unprocessed PURE BRAN
½ cup STONE-GROUND WHOLE WHEAT FLOUR
¼ cup RAW WHEAT GERM
¼ cup non-instant SKIM MILK POWDER
2 tablespoons CHIA SEEDS, ground in blender or seed grinder
1¼ teaspoons double-acting baking powder
¼ teaspoon SEA SALT

½ cup seeded, chopped DRIED PRUNES (8 large prunes)
⅔ cup warm water
1 large egg
1 tablespoon RAW HONEY
1 tablespoon BLACKSTRAP MOLASSES
¼ teaspoon baking soda
1 tablespoon COLD PRESSED ALL BLEND OIL
1 tablespoon LIQUID LECITHIN
1 teaspoon grated orange peel

Combine bran, flour, wheat germ, skim milk powder, chia seeds, baking powder and salt in a mixing bowl. (If using a food processor, blend dry ingredients with cutting blade, add seeded prunes and chop for 10 seconds.) Add prunes to mixing bowl.

In measuring cup, stir egg into water and add honey, molasses and soda. Add to dry ingredients with oil, lecithin and orange peel. Stir just to combine (5 seconds with processor).

Spoon into greased muffin tins and bake in a preheated 400 degree oven for 20 minutes, or until done.

TO MICROWAVE: Prepare batter as directed. Spoon into paper-lined microwave muffin cups. Microwave 5 at one time on full power for 2½ minutes (or until a wooden toothpick comes out clean when inserted in the center of a muffin), rotating the pan halfway through the cooking time. Repeat with the second batch of muffins.

Yield: 10 muffins

CARROT CORNBREAD

Thanks to the invisible carrots, this cornbread is deliciously moist and exceptionally high in vitamin A and potassium. Equally appetizing as corn muffins, either Carrot Cornbread or the wheat-free, yeast-leavened version which follows will complement legumes to form complete proteins for meatless meals.

¾ cup WHOLE GROUND CORNMEAL
¼ cup STONE-GROUND WHOLE WHEAT FLOUR
¼ cup non-instant SKIM MILK POWDER
¾ teaspoon SEA SALT

1 teaspoon double-acting baking powder
¾ cup warm water, divided
2 medium carrots
1 tablespoon RAW HONEY
2 tablespoons COLD PRESSED ALL BLEND OIL
2 large eggs, separated

In mixing bowl, combine cornmeal, wheat flour, skim milk powder, salt and baking powder. Scrape or peel carrots, cut in chunks and liquefy in an electric blender with ½ cup of the water. Add honey, oil and egg yolks and blend for 10 seconds. Pour the blender contents into the dry ingredients and rinse the blender with the remaining water. Stir just until mixed. Beat egg whites until stiff and fold into the batter.

Pour into an 8 × 8 × 2-inch baking pan greased with vegetable shortening. Bake in a preheated 400 degree oven for 30 minutes, or until a toothpick inserted in the center comes out clean.

TO MICROWAVE: Prepare batter as directed but use only ¾ teaspoon baking powder. Pour into an oiled 6 × 10-inch baking dish. Place on a rack or an inverted baking dish and microwave for 6 to 7 minutes (until a toothpick inserted in the center comes out clean), rotating the dish one-quarter turn each 2 minutes.

Let stand in the baking container for 5 minutes before cutting into 8 pieces.

CARROT-CORN MUFFINS:

Pour batter into greased muffin tins and bake for 20 minutes in a preheated 400 degree oven.

TO MICROWAVE: Pour batter into paper baking cups in a microwave muffin pan or individual custard cups. Place the cups in a circle and microwave half at a time for 2 minutes on full power.

Yield: 12 muffins

SUPER-NUTRITION VARIATION:

- Add with the skim milk powder:
  1 tablespoon LECITHIN GRANULES
  1 tablespoon BREWER'S YEAST
  ¼ teaspoon DOLOMITE POWDER

WHEAT-FREE YEAST CORNBREAD

¾ cup boiling water
1 teaspoon RAW HONEY
¾ cup WHOLE GROUND CORNMEAL
¼ cup warm water (115 degrees)
1½ teaspoons active dry yeast
½ cup OAT FLOUR

¼ cup non-instant SKIM MILK POWDER
½ teaspoon SEA SALT
2 tablespoons LECITHIN GRANULES
1 tablespoon COLD PRESSED ALL BLEND OIL
1 large egg

Pour boiling water into a mixing bowl and stir in honey and cornmeal. Set aside.

Sprinkle yeast over warm water in a small dish and let stand for 5 minutes, or until foamy.

Blend skim milk powder and salt into the oat flour in the measuring cup and stir into the cornmeal mixture with the lecithin granules, oil, egg, and the yeast mixture.

Pour into an 8 × 8 × 2-inch baking pan greased with vegetable shortening and let stand for 5 minutes. Bake in a preheated 400 degree oven for 25 minutes, or until a wooden toothpick inserted in the center comes out clean.

TO MICROWAVE: Combine water and honey in a glass mixing bowl. Bring to boiling in the microwave oven—about 2 minutes on full power. Stir in cornmeal and set aside. Sprinkle yeast over the ¼ cup of warm water in a small dish and let stand for 5 minutes, or until foamy.

Blend skim milk powder and salt into the oat flour in the measuring cup and stir into cornmeal mixture with lecithin granules, oil, egg, and the yeast mixture.

Pour into an oiled 6x10x2-inch baking dish and let stand for 5 minutes. Place on a rack or an inverted baking dish and microwave on full power for 5 to 6 minutes, until a toothpick inserted in the center comes out clean, rotating dish one-quarter turn each 2 minutes.

Let the cornbread stand in the pan for 5 minutes before cutting and serving.

Yield: 8 servings

WHEAT-FREE CORN MUFFINS

Pour wheat-free yeast cornbread batter into greased muffin tins and bake for 20 minutes in a preheated 400 degree oven.

TO MICROWAVE: Pour batter into paper baking cups in plastic muffin pans or individual custard cups. Place the cups in a circle and microwave half at a time for 2½ minutes on full power.

Yield: 12 small muffins

CORNBREAD COMPARISON CHART

per 1 67-gram serving, approx. 2-in. square	Homemade with enriched degermed corn-meal*	Mix made with milk*	Carrot Cornbread	Super-Nutrition Corn-bread	Wheat-free Yeast Corn-bread
Calories	150.	197.	145.	156.	155.
Protein, grams	4.75	3.0	5.0	5.76	5.8
Fiber, grams	.13	.06	.36	.36	.26
Carbohydrate, grams	23.2	34.7	19.4	20.4	21.9
Calcium, milligrams	73.	99.	87.	132.	99.
Iron, milligrams	.93	.7	.8	1.05	.95
Potassium, milligrams	105.	69.	180.	203.	165.
Vitamin A, International Units	100.	100.	1594.	1631.	252.

*from *Composition of Foods*, USDA Handbook #8

LOAF BREADS

NOTE: If it should be necessary to forego the use of electrical appliances, all of these breads may be made conventionally by replacing the electric beating, blending or processing with 10 minutes of hand kneading after the dough is mixed.

BEGINNING WHEAT BREAD

For beginning bakers as well as those who are beginning the transition from supermarket white "balloon bread" to the whole grain varieties. With electrical appliances doing the kneading, flour scooped directly from the containers without spooning, stirring, or sifting, and skim milk powder that requires no scalding, this single-rise bread can be mixed and baked in less than two hours with a conventional oven—less than one hour if a microwave oven is used to speed the rising and baking. When making future loaves, you can gradually increase the wheat-to-white-flour ratio and experiment with the variations to increase nutritional value.

1¼ cups very warm tap water
   (120 degrees)
   (cold water can be microwaved to that temperature in
   1 minute in a glass measuring
   cup)
1 tablespoon RAW HONEY
1 tablespoon active dry yeast

1¾ cups unsifted,
   UNBLEACHED WHITE
   FLOUR, divided
1 tablespoon COLD PRESSED
   ALL BLEND OIL
3 tablespoons non-instant SKIM
   MILK POWDER
1 teaspoon SEA SALT
1¼ cups STONE-GROUND
   WHOLE WHEAT FLOUR

WITH ELECTRIC BLENDER: Measure water in the blender container, add honey and mix. Sprinkle in yeast and blend on low speed for 1 second. Let stand for 5 minutes, or until foamy.

Add 1 cup of the white flour and the oil to the yeast mixture. Blend on medium speed for 30 seconds, pushing down sides each 10 seconds. Add skim milk powder and salt. Blend until the milk is dissolved, about 10 seconds, scraping down sides as needed.

Combine the remaining ¾ cup of white flour with the whole wheat flour in a mixing bowl. Stir in blender contents, kneading in the last of the flour by hand, if necessary.

WITH ELECTRIC MIXER: Combine water and honey in a mixer bowl and sprinkle yeast on the surface. Let stand 5 minutes, or until foamy.

Add 1 cup of the white flour and the oil to the yeast mixture. Beat for 3 minutes on medium speed. Add skim milk powder and salt and beat on low speed until smooth. Stir in whole wheat flour and remaining white flour, kneading in the last by hand, if necessary.

WITH FOOD PROCESSOR: Combine water and honey in the processor bowl with metal blade in place. Sprinkle yeast on the surface and let stand for 5 minutes, or until foamy.

Add 1¼ cups of the white flour and the oil. Process for 1 minute. Add skim milk powder and salt and process 5 seconds. Add remaining half-cup of white flour and the whole wheat flour. Process 5 seconds—just enough to mix in the flour, not long enough to stall the motor!

Turn out on a lightly floured sufrace and knead a few turns before shaping into a loaf.

FOR CONVENTIONAL BAKING: Place bread dough in a greased loaf pan and cover with a second, inverted loaf pan. Speed-rise by heating the oven to 100 degrees (you can check this by laying a candy thermometer on an oven rack if your oven does not have a "warm" setting), turning it off and placing the covered loaf in the oven until almost double in size. Remove bread to complete the rising and preheat the oven to 375 degrees. Remove cover and bake for approximately 35 minutes, or until crust sounds hollow when tapped.

FOR CRUSTLESS MICROWAVE BAKING: Oil a glass loaf pan. Shape the dough into a log-shaped loaf the same length as the pan. Place the loaf in the pan and cover with a second, inverted glass pan. Speed-rise by microwaving for 30 seconds on half power (Defrost setting) each 10 minutes until the dough has doubled in size—about 25 minutes. Remove cover and elevate the loaf by placing it on a microwave rack or an inverted glass baking dish. Set control on full power and microwave for 3 minutes. Turn loaf, insert microwave probe or thermometer and microwave until the internal temperature reaches 180 degrees—approximately 2 minutes. Turn the loaf out on its side on a paper towel and microwave for 30 seconds on full power to evaporate any excess moisture. Place right-side up on a rack to cool slightly before slicing.

FOR MICROWAVE BAKING PLUS A BROWNED CRUST (without a microwave browning element): Grease a glass loaf pan with vegetable shortening and/or bottom-line with a strip of parchment paper. (When baked completely with microwaves, the bread will slide right out of an oiled pan, but when conventional baking follows, it is sometimes difficult to remove the bread without gouging.) Preheat conventional oven to 400 degrees.

Shape the dough into a log-shaped loaf and place in the pan. Cover with a second, inverted loaf pan. Speed-rise by microwaving for 30 seconds on half power (Defrost setting) each 10 minutes until the dough has doubled in size—about 25 minutes. Remove cover and elevate the loaf for even baking by placing it on a microwave rack or an inverted glass baking dish. Set control on full power and microwave for 3 minutes. Turn loaf, insert microwave probe or thermometer and microwave until the internal temperature reaches 170 degrees—approximately 2 minutes. Transfer the loaf, still in the pan, to the conventional oven and bake for 10 to 15 minutes—until lightly browned. Turn out on a rack to cool slightly before slicing.

> **Toaster-oven Browning:** If the bread is microwave-baked in two small glass or ceramic pans, the loaves may be turned out of the pans before browning, so neither grease nor parchment paper need be used. Microwave both small loaves together and rearrange after 2 minutes of baking. Insert thermometer or probe and remove the bread when the internal temperature reaches 170 degrees—about 2 minutes. Brown one loaf at a time for approximately 4 minutes at 400 degrees.

VARIATIONS:

- Substitute beef, chicken or vegetable broth for the water
- Substitute LIQUID LECITHIN for the oil

- Increase the ratio of whole wheat flour to white; loaf may be made entirely with whole wheat flour
- Add 2 tablespoons GLUTEN FLOUR with the oil
- Add 1 tablespoon BREWER'S YEAST with the salt
- Substitute ¼ cup BUCKWHEAT FLOUR, OAT FLOUR, RICE FLOUR or CORNMEAL for ¼ cup of the whole wheat flour
- Blend 2 tablespoons LECITHIN GRANULES, PURE BRAN, RICE BRAN, SOY FLOUR or WHEAT GERM with the final addition of whole wheat flour
- Brush loaf with beaten egg, egg white, or milk before baking

Yield: 1½ pounds bread = 18 slices
1 large or 2 small loaves

BEGINNING RYE BREAD

1¼ cups very warm water (120 degrees)
1 tablespoon BLACKSTRAP MOLASSES
1 tablespoon active dry yeast
1¼ cups unsifted, UNBLEACHED WHITE FLOUR, divided
1 tablespoon LIQUID LECI-THIN

1 tablespoon BREWER'S YEAST
2 teaspoons caraway seeds (optional)
1 teaspoon SEA SALT
½ teaspoon grated orange peel
1¾ cups RYE FLOUR
Beaten egg or egg white for glaze

WITH ELECTRIC BLENDER: Mix water and molasses in the blender container. Sprinkle in yeast and blend on lowest speed for 1 second. Cover and let stand for 5 minutes, or until foamy.

Add 1 cup of the white flour and the lecithin to the yeast mixture. Blend on medium speed for 30 seconds, pushing down sides each 10 seconds. Add brewer's yeast, caraway seeds (if used), salt and orange peel. Blend 10 seconds.

Stir the rye flour in a mixing bowl, then stir in blender contents. Knead in the last of the white flour, if needed.

WITH ELECTRIC MIXER: Combine water and molasses in a mixer bowl and sprinkle yeast on the surface. Let stand for 5 minutes, or until foamy.

Add 1 cup of the white flour and the liquid lecithin. Beat for 3 minutes on medium speed. Add brewer's yeast, caraway seed (if used), salt and orange peel and beat for 1 minute. Stir in rye flour and knead in as much of the remaining white flour as is necessary.

WITH FOOD PROCESSOR: Combine water and molasses in the processor bowl with metal blade in place. Sprinkle yeast on the surface and let stand for 5 minutes, or until foamy.

Add the unbleached white flour and the liquid lecithin. Process for 1 minute. Add brewer's yeast, caraway seeds (if used), salt and orange peel and process for 10 seconds. Add rye flour and process until dough gathers into a ball—4 or 5 seconds.

On a lightly floured surface, shape the dough into a long, oval loaf. (If using a microwave oven, square the ends to make a log-shaped loaf.) Place in a 6 × 10-inch baking pan or dish that has been oiled and sprinkled with cornmeal. Cover and let rise to almost double. (Or speed-rise according to directions for Beginning Wheat Bread.) With a thin, sharp knife make 3 diagonal slashes in the top of the bread. Beat egg with 1 tablespoon of water and brush over the surface and into the slashes. (You can freeze the remaining egg mixture in tiny containers to use for future bakings.)

Bake as for Beginning Wheat Bread, browning the loaf if microwaves are used.

NOTE: Avoid any cornmeal clean-up by placing a sheet of waxed paper under the cooling rack before sliding the bread out of the pan to cool. Use a knife with a serrated blade or an electric knife to slice the still-warm bread.

VARIATIONS:

- Substitute beef, chicken or vegetable broth, or warm beer for the water
- Substitute WHOLE WHEAT FLOUR for all or part of the unbleached white flour
- Add 2 tablespoons GLUTEN FLOUR with the liquid lecithin
- Blend 2 tablespoons LECITHIN GRANULES, PURE BRAN, RICE BRAN, SOY FLOUR or WHEAT GERM with the rye flour.

Yield: One 22-ounce loaf = 20 slices

GOLDEN GLOW BREAD
(Carrot-wheat Blender Bread)

The carrots are noticeable only in the glowing gold color of the bread—and in the generous amounts of vitamin A and potassium they add to the other nutrients in whole-grain breads. From raw carrots to sliced bread requires less than an hour with microwaves—an hour and a half by conventional means.

½ pound carrots, peeled or scraped (1½ cups when cut in chunks)
¾ cup hot tap water (150 degrees)
1 tablespoon TURBINADO SUGAR
1 tablespoon active dry yeast

1 cup .unsifted UNBLEACHED WHITE FOUR, divided
2 tablespoons GLUTEN FLOUR
2 tablespoons SOY FLOUR
2 tablespoons COLD PRESSED ALL BLEND OIL
1 teaspoon SEA SALT
1½ cups STONE-GROUND WHOLE WHEAT FLOUR

Cut the carrots in half-inch chunks and place in a blender container with the hot water and sugar. Liquefy on high speed. Add yeast and stir in with lowest speed. (The cold carrots and hot water combine to form the ideal temperature for the yeast—115 to 120 degrees.) Let stand for 5 minutes, or until foamy.

Add one-half cup of the white flour, gluten and soy flours, oil and salt to the blender. Blend for 30 seconds on medium speed, scraping down sides once.

Combine remaining white flour with the whole wheat flour in a mixing bowl. Stir in blender contents and turn out on a floured surface. Knead for a few turns (dough will be soft and slightly sticky) and shape into a loaf. Place in a greased loaf pan, cover with a second, inverted loaf pan and let rise to double. Remove covering pan and bake in a preheated 375 degree oven for 35 minutes, or until lightly browned. Turn out on a wire cake rack to cool slightly before slicing with a serrated or electric knife.

TO MICROWAVE: Mix bread dough and shape into a loaf as directed. Place in an oiled glass loaf pan and cover with a second, inverted glass pan. Speed-rise by microwaving for 30 seconds on Defrost (half power) each 5 minutes until bread has almost doubled in size—about 15 minutes.

Remove covering pan, place loaf pan on a microwave rack and microwave on full power for 7 minutes, turning loaf twice to assure even baking. Turn loaf out on its side on a paper towel and return to the rack. Microwave 30 seconds on full power; turn over and microwave 30 seconds on the other side. Place loaf right-side up on a rack to cool slightly before slicing with a serrated or electric knife.

SUPER-NUTRITION VARIATION:

- Substitute vegetable broth for the water (or stir Vegetable Salad Powder into hot water if no broth is available)
- Substitute LIQUID LECITHIN for the All Blend Oil
- Add with the whole wheat flour: 1 tablespoon BREWER'S YEAST, ½ teaspoon DOLOMITE POWDER, ½ teaspoon B-COMPLEX POWDER

Yield: One 1½-pound loaf = 18 standard slices

RICE-BRAN WHEAT BREAD

Rice bran has a finer texture than unprocessed wheat bran, yet actually contains more fiber (11.5 grams per 100 grams, as compared to 9.1 for wheat bran). Combined with whey powder and whole grain flour it makes a delicious, basic bread—high in both fiber and protein. Slice all of the bread and freeze what is not devoured immediately, then defrost and warm meal-sized portions for a continuing supply of fresh-baked bread.

1 tablespoon active dry yeast
¼ teaspoon ground ginger
2½ cups chicken broth, homemade or canned, divided
2 tablespoons RAW HONEY
2½ cups unsifted,
  UNBLEACHED WHITE
  FLOUR
¼ cup GLUTEN FLOUR

¼ cup COLD PRESSED SAF-
  FLOWER OIL
½ cup WHEY POWDER
½ cup RICE BRAN
1¾ teaspoons SEA SALT
3½ cups STONE-GROUND
  WHOLE WHEAT FLOUR,
  not stirred

Combine yeast and ginger in a large mixing bowl. Heat broth to 115 degrees. Stir honey into 1 cup of the warm broth and pour over the yeast mixture. Let stand for 5 minutes, or until foamy.

Add remainder of broth, white flour, gluten flour, and oil. Beat on medium speed with stand mixer for 5 minutes. (Use high speed for a hand-mixer or beat 100 strokes by hand.) Using low speed, beat in whey, rice bran and salt. Stir in whole wheat flour, kneading in the last by hand. (If dough is too sticky to form a ball, add up to ¼ cup white flour.) Oil the top of the dough, cover and let rise to double. Shape into 2 loaves and place in greased loaf pans. Cover and let rise until almost double. Bake in a preheated 375 degree oven for 40 minutes (until crust sounds hollow when tapped) and turn out on a rack to cool slightly before slicing with an electric or serrated knife.

TO MICROWAVE: Place 1 cup of the chicken broth and the honey in a large glass mixing bowl. Microwave, uncovered, for 1 minute on full power—or until liquid reaches 115 degrees. Stir in ginger and sprinkle yeast on the surface. Let stand for 5 minutes, or until foamy.

Microwave remaining broth to 115 degrees in a glass

measuring cup. Add to yeast mixture with the white flour, gluten flour and oil. Beat on medium speed with stand mixer for 5 minutes. (Use high speed for a hand mixer or beat 100 strokes by hand.) Using low speed, beat in whey, rice bran and salt. Stir in whole wheat flour, kneading in the last by hand. (If dough is too sticky to form a ball, add up to ¼ cup unbleached white flour.) Oil top of dough, cover and speed-rise by microwaving on Defrost (half power) for 45 seconds each 10 minutes until the dough has doubled in size. Punch down, shape into 2 loaves and place in oiled, glass loaf pans. Speed-rise again until almost double, rearranging loaves each time they are microwaved. (If loaves remain in the microwave oven, there is no need to cover them.) Microwave both loaves together on full power for 7 minutes, rearranging twice for even baking. Transfer to a preheated, 400 degree conventional oven for 10-15 minutes—or until lightly browned. Turn out on rack to cool slightly before slicing with an electric or serrated knife.

SUPER-NUTRITION VARIATION:

- Substitute BLACKSTRAP MOLASSES for honey
- Substitute 2 tablespoons LIQUID LECITHIN for the 2 tablespoons of oil
- Add with the bran: 2 tablespoons TORULA YEAST
  1 teaspoon B-COMPLEX POWDER
  1 teaspoon DOLOMITE POWDER
  contents of 2 10,000 IU SUPER DRY A & D capsules

> **Yield: Two loaves, 1¾ pounds each**
> **36 standard slices**

SESAME EGG BREAD

A slightly irregular approach to breadmaking can pay off in savings of time and effort, without sacrificing flavor or texture. Powdered skim milk requires no scalding and the four minutes of electric-mixer beating develops the gluten even more effectively than a ten-minute hand kneading to produce a fine, elastic texture. Shaping the bread in the mixing bowl saves the bother of cleaning up a breadboard, and speeding the single rising in a warm oven saves almost half the rising time. So, even without a microwave oven, this delicious, high-protein bread can be table-ready in less than an hour and a half. If desired, double all ingredients to make two loaves.

¾ cup very warm tap water (120 degrees)

1 tablespoon RAW HONEY

1 tablespoon active dry yeast

¾ cup unsifted, UNBLEACHED WHITE FLOUR

2 tablespoons GLUTEN FLOUR

1 large egg

¼ cup SESAME SEEDS, ground in blender or seed grinder

⅓ cup non-instant SKIM MILK POWDER

1 teaspoon SEA SALT

1¼ cups STONE-GROUND WHOLE WHEAT FLOUR, not stirred

1 teaspoon whole SESAME SEEDS

Pour water into mixing bowl and stir in honey. Sprinkle on yeast and let stand for 5 minutes while assembling remaining ingredients and preparing the baking pan.

Add the unbleached white and the gluten flour and beat 4 minutes on medium speed with a stand mixer, on high speed with a hand mixer. Stir egg in measuring cup and add to the mixing bowl, reserving 1 teaspoon of the egg. Mix ground sesame seeds, skim milk powder and salt and beat in on low speed. Stir in whole wheat flour, kneading in an additional tablespoon or so, if needed, to shape into a loaf. Place in greased loaf pan. Brush with reserved egg and sprinkle with the teaspoon of sesame seeds.

Speed-rise by covering with another, inverted, loaf pan and placing in a conventional oven. Turn to ''warm'' or place a candy thermometer in the oven and turn to the lowest setting. Turn off oven when the temperature registers 100 degrees. Let bread rise until almost double. Remove and preheat oven to 375 degrees. Remove cover and bake loaf until done, about 35 minutes. Turn out on a paper towel, then place right-side up on a wire rack to cool slightly before slicing with serrated or electric knife.

TO MICROWAVE: Place water and honey in glass mixing bowl and heat to 115 degrees in the microwave oven. Prepare bread as directed and place loaf in an oiled glass loaf pan. Brush with reserved egg and sprinkle with sesame seeds. Cover with another inverted glass loaf pan and speed-rise by microwaving for 30 seconds on Defrost (half power) each 5 minutes until the loaf has doubled in size. Remove cover and place loaf in a preheated, 400 degree conventional oven for 10 minutes. (This toasts the seeds and provides a tender, lightly browned, bakery-style crust.) Transfer to the microwave oven, placing loaf on a rack or an inverted baking dish, and microwave for 4 minutes on full power—or until the internal temperature reaches 200 degrees. Turn loaf out on a paper towel, then turn right-side up on a wire rack to cool slightly before slicing with serrated or electric knife.

SUPER-NUTRITION VARIATION:

For an "irregular" instant breakfast, try a slice of this Sesame Egg Bread toasted and spread with 1 teaspoon safflower margarine and 1 tablespoon natural peanut butter. Stir ⅛ teaspoon C-Trate into your glass of juice and you're set for the morning with more protein and nourishment (and fewer calories) than you would get from an egg and a slice of regular toast with your orange juice.

- Add 1 tablespoon LIQUID LECITHIN with the gluten flour
- Add with the skim milk powder:
  1 tablespoon BREWER'S YEAST
  ½ teaspoon DOLOMITE POWDER
  ¼ teaspoon B-COMPLEX POWDER

Yield: One 20-22 ounce loaf
18 standard slices

GNC ALL-STAR BREAD

Thanks to "All-Star 95% Protein Supreme" this is THE BREAD for carbohydrate counters, cholesterol dodgers, low-blood-sugar-dieters, and weight watchers—each medium-sized loaf contains as much protein as 18 eggs (without the cholesterol), more calcium and magnesium than a quart of whole milk (without the fat and calories), and the blackstrap and brewer's yeast combine with the whole grain wheat to provide iron, B-vitamins and potassium . . . all in this delicious, non-crumbly, easy-mix, single rise bread. Low-sodium dieters can omit the salt and still have the satisfying flavor of real bread because of the seasonings in the broth, and either version has the unbelievably amazing protein-carbohydrate ratio of more than six grams of protein to less than ten grams of carbohydrate per slice.

ALL-STAR PROTEIN BREAD #1
(2 loaves, made with electric mixer)

1 cup *each* beef and chicken broth, homemade or canned, warmed to 115 degrees

2 teaspoons BLACKSTRAP MOLASSES

3 tablespoons active dry yeast

1 cup GLUTEN FLOUR

½ cup unsifted UNBLEACHED WHITE FLOUR

3 tablespoons LIQUID LECITHIN

⅔ cup non-instant SKIM MILK POWDER

3 ounces (6 heaping tablespoons) ALL-STAR 95% PROTEIN SUPREME POWDER

3 tablespoons BREWER'S YEAST

1 teaspoon DOLOMITE POWDER

1¼ teaspoons SEA SALT

1⅓ cups STONE-GROUND WHOLE WHEAT FLOUR

1 medium egg white

In a large mixer bowl, stir molasses into broth, sprinkle yeast on the surface and let stand for 5 minutes, or until foamy.

Stir in gluten flour, white flour and lecithin. Beat for 5 minutes on medium speed with a stand mixer, on high speed with a portable mixer. Combine skim milk powder, protein powder, brewer's yeast, dolomite and salt. Stir into dough until thoroughly mixed, or beat in with dough hooks on low speed. Stir in wheat flour and turn out on a lightly floured surface. Knead just enough to shape into 2 medium loaves and place in greased pans. Brush with egg white beaten with ½ teaspoon water, cover and let rise until just barely double in size. (Allowing the bread to rise too much can result in "fallen loaves" which are edible, but not too attractive.) Bake loaves in a preheated 375 degree oven for 35 minutes, or until done. Turn out on a wire rack to cool slightly before slicing with an electric or serrated knife.

TO MICROWAVE: Make and shape bread dough and let rise as directed. Use oiled glass loaf pans and microwave one loaf at a time. Place loaf on a rack and microwave 4½ minutes on full power, turning after 3 minutes. (Internal temperature should reach 180 degrees.) Turn out on a paper towel and return to the microwave, if necessary, for 30 seconds to dry any excess moisture on the bottom and sides. If desired, the microwaved loaves may be browned under a microwave browner, or left in their pans and browned for 10 minutes in a 400 degree conventional oven.

Yield: Two 18-ounce loaves
36 standard slices

ALL-STAR PROTEIN BREAD #2
(1 loaf, made with food processor)

1 cup chicken broth, homemade or canned, warmed to 115 degrees

1 teaspoon BLACKSTRAP MOLASSES

1½ tablespoons active dry yeast

½ cup GLUTEN FLOUR

⅓ cup unsifted UNBLEACHED WHITE FLOUR

1½ tablespoons LIQUID LECITHIN

⅓ cup non-instant SKIM MILK POWDER

1½ ounces (3 heaping tablespoons) ALL-STAR 95% PROTEIN SUPREME

1½ tablespoons BREWER'S YEAST

¾ teaspoon SEA SALT

½ teaspoon DOLOMITE POWDER

¾ cup STONE-GROUND WHOLE WHEAT FLOUR

Combine broth and molasses in the processor bowl with

metal blade in place. Sprinkle yeast on the surface and let stand 5 minutes, or until foamy.

Add gluten flour, white flour and lecithin and process for 1 minute. Add skim milk powder, protein powder, brewer's yeast, salt and dolomite and process for 5 seconds. Add whole wheat flour and process until mixture gathers into a ball—5 to 10 seconds.

Turn dough out on a lightly floured surface and knead just enough to shape into a loaf. Place in a greased loaf pan, cover and let rise until just barely double in size; over-rising will cause the bread to fall.

Bake conventionally for 35 minutes in a preheated 375 degree oven and turn out on a wire rack.

> **TO MICROWAVE:** Prepare dough and let rise as directed, using a glass loaf pan. Microwave on a rack for 4½ minutes on full power, turning loaf after 3 minutes. Brown, if desired, as for All-Star Bread #1.

**Yield: 1 medium loaf
18 standard slices**

TENDER-CRUST ROLLS

Made on the order of puff pastry (but with much less time and bother), this super-nutritious, flaky-tender roll dough may be shaped as French croissants, cut for Fan Tans, or spread with Honey-Butter to make breakfast sweet rolls.

1¼ cups very warm water (120 degrees)
1 tablespoon RAW BROWN SUGAR
1 tablespoon active dry yeast
1½ cups unsifted UNBLEACHED WHITE FLOUR
¼ cup non-instant SKIM MILK POWDER
2 tablespoons RAW HONEY
1 tablespoon LIQUID LECITHIN

2 tablespoons toasted WHEAT GERM
1 tablespoon BREWER'S YEAST
1 teaspoon SEA SALT
1¼ cups plus 2 tablespoons STONE-GROUND WHOLE WHEAT FLOUR
½ cup safflower margarine, at room temperature
1 large egg
1 tablespoon milk

Stir brown sugar into the water in a mixing bowl and sprinkle yeast on the surface. Let stand for 5 minutes, or until foamy.

Combine white flour with skim milk powder in the measuring cup and add to the yeast mixture with the honey and lecithin. Beat with an electric mixer for 3 minutes on medium speed. Stir wheat germ, brewer's yeast and salt into the 1¼ cups of whole wheat flour, then stir into the dough. Turn out on the remaining 2 tablespoons of whole wheat flour and knead two or three turns to make a smooth ball.

Roll or pat to a 10-inch square. Spread margarine on all but a 3-inch strip across one side and a 1-inch margin on the ends. Fold the bare strip of dough over half the margarine, then fold the remaining margarine-spread dough over the top to make a rectangle approximately 4 × 10-inches. Pinch edges to seal in the margarine and gently roll to a thickness of ¾-inch. Fold in thirds, cover with a sheet of waxed paper and let stand for 10 minutes. Repeat rolling and folding once more, then place the dough in a covered bowl in the refrigerator for 1 or 2 hours.

For Croissants—Crescent Rolls: Cut the chilled dough in half. Without kneading, gently roll each half into a 12-inch circle on a lightly floured surface. Cut each circle into 8 pie-shaped sections and roll each section from the base to the tip. Place on a greased baking sheet with the points down to hold them in place. Curve the ends to form crescents. Beat the egg and milk together and brush over each roll. Let rise until double, about 30 minutes, and brush again. Bake in a preheated 400 degree oven for 15 minutes, or until lightly browned.

Yield: 16 crescent rolls

For Fan Tans: Turn the chilled dough out onto a

lightly floured surface and, without kneading, gently pat and roll to ¼-inch thickness. Spread thinly with additional soft margarine (about 1 tablespoon) and cut into 1½-inch strips, then cut across the strips to make 1½-inch squares. Stack four squares together and place them on end in a greased muffin cup. Repeat with remaining squares to make 16 fan tan rolls. Whisk together egg and milk and brush the tops of the rolls. Let rise until double in size, about 30 minutes, brush again with the beaten egg and bake in a preheated 400 degree oven for 15 minutes, or until lightly browned.

Yield: 16 rolls

VARIATION: *CINNAMON-HONEY BREAKFAST ROLLS*

Tender-Crust Roll dough
¼ cup Honey Butter (recipe on page 152)
¼ cup RAW BROWN SUGAR, firmly packed
½ teaspoon cinnamon
Sugar Glaze (optional) recipe follows

Turn the chilled dough out on a lightly floured surface. Without kneading, gently roll and pat to a ¼-inch thick rectangle. Spread with honey-butter, then sprinkle with brown sugar and cinnamon. Cut in half to make two 9 × 12-inch sections. Roll jelly-roll fashion to form two 12-inch logs. Cut each into 12 pieces, flatten each to a 2½-inch circle and arrange one-half inch apart on a greased baking sheet. Do *not* brush with egg and milk. Let rise until double and bake in a preheated 400 degree oven for 15 minutes, or until lightly browned.

Optional SUGAR GLAZE: If desired, make confectioners sugar by processing or blending turbinado sugar until it is powdery. Blend ¾ cup of the "powdered" sugar with 1 tablespoon water and ⅛ teaspon vanilla. Drizzle over warm rolls.

Yield: 24 rolls

SANDWICH BUNS OR ROLLS

With a supply of these rolls in the freezer, you're prepared for instant and nutritious meals.

1 cup warm water (115 degrees)
1 tablespoon RAW HONEY
1 tablespoon active dry yeast
2 tablespoons COLD PRESSED ALL BLEND OIL
1 tablespoon LIQUID LECITHIN
2 cups unsifted UNBLEACHED WHITE FLOUR, divided

⅓ cup non-instant SKIM MILK POWDER
2 tablespoons SOY FLOUR
1 tablespoon BREWER'S YEAST
1½ teaspoons SEA SALT
2 large egg whites
2 tablespoons toasted WHEAT GERM
1 cup STONE-GROUND WHOLE WHEAT FLOUR

WITH ELECTRIC MIXER: Combine water and honey in mixer bowl. Sprinkle active dry yeast on the surface and let stand for 5 minutes, or until foamy.

Add oil, lecithin and 1 cup of the white flour. Beat on medium speed for 4 minutes. Stir skim milk powder, soy flour, brewer's yeast and salt in the measuring cup and stir into the batter with the egg whites and wheat germ. Beat on medium speed until thoroughly blended. Stir in whole wheat flour and remaining white flour, kneading in the last of the flour by hand. Shape into a ball and turn in an oiled bowl.

WITH FOOD PROCESSOR: Combine water and honey in processor bowl with metal blade. Sprinkle active dry yeast on the surface and let stand for 5 minutes, or until foamy.

Add oil, liquid lecithin and 1¼ cups of the white flour. Process for 1 minute. Add skim milk powder, soy flour, brewer's yeast, salt and egg whites and process for 10 seconds. Add remaining white flour, wheat germ and whole wheat flour. Process for 5 seconds, or until mixture gathers into a ball. Turn out into an oiled bowl and shape into a smooth ball.

Cover bowl and let dough rise until double in size—about 1 hour. Punch down and divide into 12 balls for medium-sized rolls, 8 balls for large rolls. Shape each ball into a round, half-inch-thick bun or 5-inch long roll and place on a cookie sheet greased with vegetable shortening. Cover and let rise until almost double in size. Bake in a preheated 400 degree oven for 12 minutes, or until lightly browned.

TO MICROWAVE: Speed-rise the covered bowl of dough by microwaving on Defrost (half power) for 30 seconds each 5 minutes until the dough has doubled in size—about 20 minutes. Divide dough into 8 or 12 pieces and shape into buns or rolls. Place buns on strips of parchment paper on a microwave baking dish or a piece of cardboard. Cover and let rise until almost double. Microwave 4 large or 6 medium buns for 3 minutes on full power, turning dish after 2 minutes. If desired, brown under a microwave browning unit or in a hot conventional oven.

FOR TOPPINGS: Brush the shaped rolls with egg or egg white beaten with a little water and sprinkle with sesame or poppy seeds.

SUPER-NUTRITION VARIATION:

- Reduce unbleached white flour to 1¼ cups
- Increase stone-ground whole wheat flour to 1¾ cups
- Add ¼ teaspoon B-COMPLEX POWDER and ¼ teaspoon DOLOMITE POWDER with the skim milk powder

Yield: 8 large or 12 medium rolls

TO FREEZE BAKED ROLLS:

Cool rolls on wire racks and quick-freeze by placing the racks in the coldest part of the freezer. Package on styrofoam trays or paper plates inside plastic bags. Defrost and warm in the microwave oven, or transfer to a metal pan and warm in a conventional oven.

TO FREEZE BROWN & SERVE ROLLS

With conventional oven: Remove rolls from the oven before they are browned—after about 13 minutes of baking. Cool, package and freeze. When ready to serve, place the frozen rolls on a baking sheet and bake for approximately 8 minutes in a 400 degree oven. Glaze the Cinnamon-Honey Rolls after the final baking.

With microwave oven: Your microwave oven can save both time and energy with the preliminary baking of your own brown and serve rolls. Many of the bread recipes are suitable for dinner rolls (Golden Glow or Sesame Egg Bread, Tender-Crust Rolls or Sandwich Buns are especially appealing), and a pan of rolls can go from the freezer to the table with only a ten-minute browning in a hot oven.

Instead of shaping the breads or rolls as directed, form the dough into round or oval rolls and place them in a circle on a microwave baking sheet or in an 8 or 9-inch round baking dish. Brush with softened margarine and sprinkle with sesame or poppy seeds. Cover and let rise until doubled in size. Microwave on full power for 3½-4 minutes (until no longer doughy) rotating the dish once or twice. Remove from the baking pan and allow to cool before wrapping and freezing. When ready to serve, place the frozen rolls on a cookie sheet and bake in a preheated 425 degree oven for 8 to 10 minutes.

STEAMED BROWN BREAD

This yeast-leavened version of Boston Brown Bread exemplifies combining great taste and eye appeal with good nutrition. It is exceptionally low in sodium and high in iron and potassium and has over 2½ grams of protein to 11 grams of carbohydrate in each 54-calorie slice. Even without the traditional accompaniment of baked beans, these round slices are substantial enough to serve as a complete snack-meal with a spread, salad or fruit, and a beverage. If you have a microwave oven, by all means take advantage of its super-quick steaming ability.

¼ cup YELLOW CORNMEAL	¼ cup SOY FLOUR
1 cup boiling water	1 tablespoon BREWER'S
¼ cup warm water (115 degrees)	YEAST
1 tablespoon active dry yeast	½ teaspoon SEA SALT
½ cup STONE-GROUND	¼ cup BLACKSTRAP
WHOLE WHEAT FLOUR	MOLASSES
½ cup RYE FLOUR	½ cup seedless RAISINS
⅓ cup non-instant SKIM MILK	
POWDER	

Gradually stir cornmeal into boiling water in a mixing bowl and let stand.

Sprinkle yeast on warm water in a small bowl and let stand 5 minutes.

In a 4-cup measure, combine the whole wheat flour, rye flour, skim milk powder, soy flour, brewer's yeast and salt, blending with a whisk or fork.

Stir molasses into the cornmeal then stir in combined dry ingredients and the yeast mixture. Beat with a spoon until smooth, then stir in raisins.

TO STEAM IN A KETTLE: Grease three 14 to 16-ounce fruit or vegetable cans with vegetable shortening and spoon in the batter, filling each one approximately half full. Cover cans with squares of greased aluminum foil and press down sides to seal. Place on a rack in a deep kettle and pour in hot water to come two inches up the sides of the cans. Cover kettle and bring water to boiling over medium heat. Lower heat and simmer, covered, for 2 hours—or until a toothpick inserted in the center of a bread comes out clean. Invert the cans on a cutting board for 5 minutes. If bread has not dropped down in the cans, open the ends with a can opener and push out the breads.

TO PRESSURE STEAM: Grease three 14 to 16-ounce fruit or vegetable cans with vegetable shortening and spoon in the batter, filling each one just over half full. Cover cans with squares of greased aluminum foil and press down sides to seal. Place on a rack in the pressure cooker with water 1-inch deep around the cans. Cover with lid but do not put pressure control in place. Bring to boiling, then reduce heat and cook for 15 minutes with steam escaping through the vent pipe. Put pressure control in place and cook for 20 minutes after full pressure is reached. Let pressure drop of its own accord. Remove foil covering and invert cans on a cutting board for 5 minutes. If bread has not dropped down in the cans, open the ends with a can opener and push out the breads.

TO STEAM WITH MICROWAVES: Oil three 1-pint wide-mouth jars and spoon in the batter, filling each one approximately half full. Cover the jars with plastic wrap and secure with rubber bands. Place in the microwave oven with an uncovered jar or cup of water and set control on Defrost (half power). Microwave for 16 to 18 minutes, rearranging jars each 5 minutes. (Breads should be pulling away from the sides of the jars at the top and a toothpick inserted in the center of a bread should come out clean.) Remove covers and invert jars on a cutting board until the breads slide down, then slowly lift jars up and away from the breads.

NOTE: Ceramic cheese crocks, with their bails removed, make wonderful steaming containers, when their own lids are used instead of plastic wrap. (Before using the crocks, test them for microwave use: Place a crock in a casserole, half fill the crock with water and pour water in the casserole to the depth of 1 inch. Microwave on full power for 1 minute. The water should be warm and the upper half of the crock should be cool.) The cooled, sliced bread can be kept in the refrigerator in the washed crocks—with the bails replaced for airtight covering.

Yield: 21 ounces = 21 slices

VARIATION: *STEAMED DATE-NUTBREAD*

Adding dates and nuts increases the quantity as well as the healthful nutrients, and makes a lusciously rich-tasting dessert without eggs, sugar or oil.

1 cup boiling water
2 tablespoons RAW HONEY
¼ cup YELLOW CORNMEAL
1 tablespoon active dry yeast
¼ cup warm water (115 degrees)
½ cup STONE-GROUND WHOLE WHEAT FLOUR
½ cup RYE FLOUR
⅓ cup non-instant SKIM MILK POWDER
¼ cup SOY FLOUR

2 tablespoons WHEAT GERM
1 tablespoon BREWER'S YEAST
½ teaspoon SEA SALT
¼ cup BLACKSTRAP MOLASSES
1 cup chopped DATES, firmly packed
½ cup chopped walnuts
¼ cup LECITHIN GRANULES

Combine boiling water and honey in a mixing bowl, then gradually stir in the cornmeal. Let stand.

Sprinkle yeast on warm water in a small bowl and let stand 5 minutes, or until foamy.

In a 4-cup measure, combine the whole wheat flour, rye flour, dry milk, soy flour, wheat germ, brewer's yeast and salt, blending with a whisk or fork.

Stir molasses into the cornmeal mixture, then stir in combined dry ingredients and the yeast mixture. Beat with a spoon until smooth, then stir in dates, nuts and lecithin granules.

Steam as for Steamed Brown Bread, using 4 containers instead of three, if needed to have them no more than half full, and allowing an additional 5 minutes of microwaving time.

Yield: 30 ounces = 30 slices

CHAPTER 8

Desserts

ICE CREAM & FROZEN DESSERTS
PUDDINGS, PIE FILLINGS
& FROZEN DESSERTS
PIES
CAKES, FILLINGS,
FROSTINGS & TOPPINGS
COOKIES & CANDIES

OLD-FASHIONED CUSTARD ICE CREAM

Rich and smooth, yet calorie and carbohydrate reduced (note comparison chart) and easily prepared in a refrigerator-freezer. Adding gelatin to improve the texture (and increase the protein) isn't a new idea—it's been done in our family for 80 years—but skim milk powder and liquid lecithin are definitely modern improvements.

½ cup non-instant SKIM MILK POWDER
⅓ cup TURBINADO SUGAR
2 tablespoons FRUCTOSE GRANULES
1 tablespoon PURE GELATIN
½ teaspoon DOLOMITE POWDER
⅛ teaspoon SEA SALT

¾ cup warm water
2 large eggs
1 tablespoon LIQUID LECITHIN
¾ cup ice water
1½ teaspoons pure vanilla
1 cup heavy cream
⅛ teaspoon C-TRATE

In a small mixer bowl, combine skim milk powder, sugar, fructose, gelatin, dolomite and salt. Gradually add water, beating until smooth. Beat in eggs and pour into a saucepan. Cook and stir over low heat until the mixture is beginning to simmer around the edges.

TO MICROWAVE: Leave the mixture in the glass mixer bowl and microwave on full power until beginning to simmer around the edges—about 3 minutes—stirring once each minute.

Beat in lecithin, ice water and vanilla. Transfer to a metal pan (or leave in the mixing bowl if there is room in the freezer) and freeze until partially frozen.

Whip cream and C-Trate and set aside. Beat the frosty mixture until creamy, then fold in the whipped cream and pour into freezer containers. Cover and freeze until solid.

NOTE: For a frozen custard effect, allow the ice cream to soften in the refrigerator for a few minutes before serving.

Yield: 5 cups
Ten ½-cup servings

ALMOST ICE CREAM

A delightful way to enjoy the benefits of the illusive vitamin U (the anti-ulcer vitamin) which is present in raw egg yolks and raw, unheated milk. Now that scientific tests have shown that small amounts of raw egg white won't harm the B vitamins, the only heating required is for dissolving the gelatin and destroying the enzymes in uncooked soy flour which can block the utilization of micronutrients and the absorption of protein. The flavor and texture equal those of commercial ice cream, with fewer calories and carbohydrates plus more protein and calcium—see the comparison chart following the recipe.

1½ cups water, including 2 ice cubes, divided
⅓ cup TURBINADO SUGAR
2 tablespoons SOY FLOUR
1 tablespoon PURE GELATIN
⅛ teaspoon SEA SALT
⅔ cup non-instant SKIM MILK POWDER
2 tablespoons safflower margarine

1 tablespoon LIQUID LECITHIN
1 cup raw, whole milk
2 large eggs, separated
2 teaspoons LIQUID SUBSTI-SWEET
1½ teaspoons pure vanilla
1 large egg white
⅛ teaspoon C-TRATE

Measure ¾ cup water in the container of an electric blender. Combine sugar, soy flour, gelatin and salt with the dry milk and blend with the water on medium speed. Pour into a small saucepan. Cook and stir until simmering.

TO MICROWAVE: Pour into a 2-cup glass measure and microwave on full power for 2 minutes.

Return to the blender container, add margarine and lecithin and blend on high speed for 10 seconds. Add remaining water with 1 ice cube, the milk, egg yolks, Substi-Sweet and vanilla. Blend on high speed for one minute. Add the last ice cube and blend on high speed until the ice is dissolved. Pour into a metal bowl or pan and place in the freezer until thickened (one or two hours). Beat egg whites with C-Trate until stiff but not dry. Process or beat the frosty mixture until smooth, then fold into the egg whites. Transfer to freezer containers and freeze until solid.

Yield: Ten ½-cup servings

COMPARISON CHART

	Almost Ice Cream	*Old-Fashioned Custard Ice Cream*	*Commercial Ice Milk**	*Commercial Ice Cream**
per ½ cup				
Calories	124.2	164.9	144.5	194.5
Protein, grams	6.2	4.7	4.5	3.7
Fats, grams	5.6	11.2	4.9	12.0
Carbohydrates, grams	12.4	11.7	21.5	19.5
Calcium, milligrams	169.0	145.0	148.0	115.0

---

*from *Nutrition Almanac*, McGraw Hill Paperbacks, 1975.

CARAMEL PUDDING

A microwave oven is worth its counter space just for making puddings. If you have a microwave, by all means use it. If not, utilize the same, one-pan method for stove-top cooking and leave the double-cooker in the cupboard. Adding vitamin A and D to the powdered milk ''enriches'' it much as the dairies do, and contributes to the impressive nutritional score for this dessert (see the analysis tables).

⅔ cup RAW BROWN SUGAR
⅓ cup non-instant SKIM MILK POWDER
contents of 1 10,000 IU SUPER DRY VITAMIN A & D capsule
3 tablespoons ARROWROOT or cornstarch
2 tablespoons SOY FLOUR
¼ teaspoon SEA SALT

1¾ cups warm water
1 large egg
1 tablespoon BLACKSTRAP MOLASSES
2 tablespoons safflower margarine
1 tablespoon LIQUID LECITHIN
½ teaspoon PURE VANILLA

Mix sugar, dry milk, vitamin A & D from the capsule, arrowroot, soy flour and salt in a medium saucepan. Gradually add water, stirring to keep smooth. Whisk in egg and molasses. Cook and stir over low heat for 12 to 15 minutes, stirring constantly during the last few minutes to prevent sticking. Remove from heat as soon as pudding is thickened and beginning to bubble.

TO MICROWAVE: Mix sugar, skim milk powder, vitamin A & D from the capsule, soy flour, arrowroot and salt in a 4-cup glass measure. Gradually add water, stirring to keep smooth. Whisk in egg and molasses. Microwave, uncovered, for 4 minutes on full power. Stir after 2 minutes, then leave the wooden stirring spoon in the pudding and stir twice more. Remove as soon as the pudding is thickened and beginning to bubble.

Add margarine, lecithin and vanilla. Whisk in until smooth. For professional smoothness and texture, pour the hot pudding into an electric blender container or processor work bowl and blend in the margarine, lecithin and vanilla.

Pour into serving dishes and refrigerate until cool. Serve with a dollop of whipped topping, if desired.

VARIATIONS:

● *Caramel-Carob Pudding*—Stir ¼ cup CAROB CHIPS into the warm pudding (without completely melting the chips) before pouring into serving dishes.

• *Caramel-Banana Pudding*—Slice 1 large banana and stir into the warm pudding before pouring into serving dishes.

NOTE FOR THOSE WHO NEED EXTRA CALCIUM: Add 1 teaspoon DOLOMITE POWDER and ½ teaspoon BONE MEAL POWDER with the dry ingredients. This will provide the equivalent of more than two 8-ounce glasses of milk in each half-cup serving of pudding.

Yield: 4 servings

NECTARINE-GRAPE MOUSSE

Delectably palate-cleansing and refreshing, with no tell-tale tang of yogurt. . . . serve on crisp greens as a fruit salad or create a low-calorie dessert with pizzaz by garnishing with additional grapes, slices of fresh nectarine and dollops of whipped topping.

1 tablespoon PURE GELATIN	½ cup ACIDOPHILUS YOGURT
½ cup orange juice	2 cups chopped fresh nectarines, with peelings
2 tablespoons RAW HONEY	½ cup seedless, green grapes
⅛ teaspoon ground allspice	
1/16 teaspoon SEA SALT	

Sprinkle gelatin on orange juice and let stand for 5 minutes. Heat and stir to dissolve gelatin. (Use a small saucepan for stove-top, a glass measuring cup for 1 minute of microwaving.) Stir in honey, allspice and salt.

Measure yogurt in blender container, add nectarines and puree until smooth. Add gelatin mixture and blend. Pour into a 3 or 4 cup container and chill until mixture mounds on a spoon. Stir in grapes, cut in half if large, and transfer to 1 large or 6 small molds. Chill several hours before serving.

VARIATION: When nectarines aren't in season, substitute drained, canned peaches or apricots, packed in their own juice, and use it in place of the orange juice. "Fresh" grapes are always available if you keep a bag of frozen ones in the freezer.

SUPER-NUTRITION VARIATION:

- Add to the nectarines before pureeing:
  1 tablespoon BREWER'S YEAST
  ¼ teaspoon C-TRATE
  contents of 1 10,000 IU SUPER DRY A & D capsule

Yield: 6 servings

SULTAN'S DELIGHT
(fig pudding)

Satisfyingly rich, yet light tasting and refreshing, this fabulous dessert has an amazing amount of protein, fiber, vitamins, minerals . . . and some well-camouflaged yogurt. Temperature is the key to full nutritional benefits—the helpful acidophilus in the yogurt are unharmed when the pudding temperature is allowed to drop to 120 degrees before it is added.

1 tablespoon WHOLE WHEAT PASTRY FLOUR	1 medium egg white
½ cup water	¼ teaspoon SEA SALT
3 tablespoons RAW HONEY	1 cup ACIDOPHILUS YOGURT
½ cup NATURAL CASHEW BUTTER	½ cup CAROB NUGGETS (or three 1-ounce CAROB BARS, grated or chopped)
¾ cup chopped DRIED FIGS	

Blend flour and water in a 2-quart saucepan. Stir in honey and cook until thickened, stirring frequently. Stir in cashew butter and figs. Cook and stir over low heat until simmering. Remove from heat and fold in the egg white which has been stiffly beaten with the salt. Let stand to cool to 120 degrees before adding the yogurt and carob. (Hasten the cooling by placing the pan in a larger bowl of ice cubes and water.) Chill before serving, embellished with whipped topping, if desired.

TO MICROWAVE: Blend flour and water in a 4-cup glass measure. Stir in honey and microwave for 3 minutes, stirring once. Stir in cashew butter and figs. Cover and microwave until simmering—about 3 minutes—stirring once. Beat egg white with the salt until it stands in stiff peaks, then fold into the pudding mixture. Let stand for a few minutes (or cool in a bowl of ice cubes and water) so the temperature will go down to 120 degrees before stirring in the yogurt and carob pieces. Chill before serving in individual dishes, embellished with whipped topping, if desired.

NOTE: For a smoother texture, transfer the simmering pudding to a processor work bowl with the cutting blade in place. Process for 10 seconds before blending with the egg white.

Yield: Six ½-cup servings

HONEY-BAKED PEARS

Naturally delicious and packed with vitamins instead of calories.

2 tablespoons water
1 tablespoon RAW HONEY
⅛ teaspoon C-TRATE
¼ cup seedless RAISINS

¼ cup finely chopped walnuts
1 tablespoon WHEAT GERM
2 large, ripe pears (¾ pound)

Combine water, honey and C-Trate in a small dish and set aside.

Blend raisins, walnuts and wheat germ with 1 tablespoon of the honey mixture and set aside.

Cut pears in half and core. Remove peelings only if they are very tough. Firmly mound one-fourth of the raisin mixture on each pear half and arrange them in a baking dish or casserole. Spoon the remainder of the honey mixture over the pears and filling. Cover with a lid or aluminum foil and bake in a preheated 350 degree oven for 30 minutes. (Or microwave for 4 minutes on full power in a baking dish covered with a lid or plastic wrap.) Spoon the cooking liquid over the pears and serve warm or cold.

Yield: 4 servings

VARIATION: *SNOW-CAPPED PEARS*

A special dessert with little fat and no starch. To serve warm without last-minute bother, bake the pears and make the sauce the day before serving. Cover with the beaten egg whites and warm the sauce while the meringue is baking.

1 recipe Honey-Baked Pears	2 tablespoons COCONUT MEAL
2 egg whites	2 1-ounce CAROB BARS,
2 tablespoons RAW BROWN SUGAR	chopped or grated or ⅓ cup CAROB NUGGETS

Prepare, fill and bake pears as directed but reduce the cooking time to 20 minutes in the conventional oven, 3 minutes in the microwave. Lift pears to an oven-proof serving dish (or dishes) and reserve the cooking liquid. (If there is more than ¼ cup of liquid, reduce it by boiling.)

Beat egg whites until frothy and gradually beat in the brown sugar, beating until thick and glossy. Fold in the coconut and swirl over the top and sides of each pear half. Reduce conventional oven heat to 300 degrees and bake for 15 minutes, or microwave for 5 minutes on the Defrost setting (half power).

Heat the reserved liquid to boiling and stir in the carob, stirring until smooth. Drizzle over the meringue-topped pears and serve warm or cold.

Yield: 4 servings

FROZEN DESSERT CREPES

Delightfully refreshing for a summer dessert or snack; freeze a supply of these crepes when fresh fruits are plentiful and hoard a few for an unexpected treat on Indian Summer days in the fall. High in vitamin A, potassium and iron, their high-protein, low-fat and low-calorie content qualifies them as weight-watcher fare. Honeydew melon and/or fresh peaches may be substituted for the cantaloupe and nectarines if the contents of a Super Dry Vitamin A & D capsule is sprinkled in with the fructose. (Nectarines have more potassium and vitamin A than peaches, while one-half cup of cantaloupe contains 2020 more International Units of vitamin A than an equal amount of either honeydew or casaba melon.)

1 cup diced, ripe nectarines
1 medium banana, diagonally sliced
½ cup diced cantaloupe
1 teaspoon FRUCTOSE GRANULES
¼ teaspoon C-TRATE
½ cup fresh or unsweetened, frozen blueberries

½ cup ACIDOPHILUS YOGURT
2 tablespoons ORANGE BLOSSOM HONEY
½ teaspoon freshly grated orange peel*
6 Basic Crepes (recipe on page 169)

Peel nectarines only if the skin is tough or blemished. Combine with banana and cantaloupe in a mixing bowl and sprinkle with fructose and C-Trate. Toss to combine and add blueberries.

Stir honey and orange peel into yogurt and blend one half of the mixture with the fruit. Spread one-third cup of the fruit mixture on each crepe and roll up as for a jelly roll. Place seam-sides down on a flat pan and spoon remaining yogurt sauce over the tops. Quick-freeze on the pan, then transfer to a styrofoam tray or paper plates before wrapping for freezer storage. Refrigerate for a few minutes to partially defrost before serving.

*To arrange for year-round fresh orange peel: freeze the rinds from juiced oranges and grate them as needed—the grating is much easier than with fresh oranges and the flavor is the same.

Yield: 6 servings of 1 crepe each

WHEAT PASTRY

Quickly and easily prepared, this polyunsaturated pastry, with its nut-like flavor, requires no chilling before rolling.

1 cup STONE-GROUND WHOLE WHEAT FLOUR
½ cup unsifted, UNBLEACHED WHITE FLOUR

1 tablespoon RAW WHEAT GERM
1 tablespoon LECITHIN GRANULES

½ teaspoon SEA SALT
¼ teaspoon B-COMPLEX POW-
DER (optional)
6 tablespoons COLD PRESSED
SAFFLOWER OIL

2 tablespoons COLD PRESSED
WALNUT OIL
3 or 4 tablespoons cold water

Combine flours, wheat germ, lecithin, salt and B-complex powder (if used) in a mixing bowl. Stir in oils with a fork and add water until mixture can be formed into a ball.

WITH FOOD PROCESSOR: Place dry ingredients in processor bowl with cutting blade in place and process for 3 on/off turns or pulsations. Add oils and process 10 seconds. With processor running normally, add water through the feed tube until mixture gathers into a ball.

FOR 2 PASTRY SHELLS: Divide mixture into 2 balls and roll to 12-inch circles between sheets of waxed paper. Line two 9-inch pie plates, prick with a fork and flute edges. Bake in a preheated 400 degree oven for 12 to 15 minutes.

TO MICROWAVE: Prepare as directed, using glass pie plates. Microwave one shell at a time for 4½ minutes on full power, rotating one-quarter turn each 1½ minutes. (Elevating the pie plate on a rack or a second, inverted pie plate and placing it off-center in the oven will assure even baking.)

FOR DOUBLE CRUSTS: Follow individual recipe directions.

Note: When you need only one pastry shell, the remaining half of the dough can be refrigerated for several days or frozen for longer storage.

CHUNKY PINEAPPLE-PEAR PUDDING OR PIE FILLING

A quick-fix, vitamin-packed dessert that is light on calories and heavy on protein—especially when you include All-Star 95%

Protein Supreme. Substitute canned pears when fresh ones aren't in season and serve at any time of year for the finishing touch to a perfect meal.

1 tablespoon PURE GELATIN	1½ tablespoons FRUCTOSE
½ cup water	GRANULES
1 8-ounce can chunk pineapple	2 large, ripe pears (¾ pound)
in its own juice	1 large egg
⅓ cup non-instant SKIM MILK	¼ teaspoon C-TRATE
POWDER	3 ice cubes

Sprinkle gelatin on the water in a small saucepan and let stand for 5 minutes. Heat and stir to dissolve. (Or microwave in a glass measuring cup for 1½ minutes on full power.) Pour into the container of an electric blender.

Drain pineapple and add the juice to the hot gelatin mixture with the skim milk powder and fructose. Blend for 5 seconds. Core pears and remove peelings if coarse or blemished. Chop 1 pear and add to blender with egg, C-Trate, and 1 ice cube. Blend on high speed for 10 seconds; add the second ice cube and blend 10 seconds. Add the final ice cube and blend until all the ice has melted.

Dice remaining pear and stir into the pudding with the pineapple. Pour into serving dishes and chill until set—about 30 minutes.

SUGAR-FREE VARIATION:

● Substitute 1⅛ teaspoon SUBSTI-SWEET for the fructose granules

(This super-nutrition variation with Substi-Sweet has 100 calories per serving, 18 grams of carbohydrate and 9.5 grams of protein.)

SUPER-NUTRITION VARIATION:

● Add with the dry milk: 1 ounce ALL-STAR 95% PRO-TEIN SUPREME
contents of 1 10,000 IU SUPER DRY A & D capsule

¼ teaspoon DOLOMITE
POWDER

VARIATION: *PINEAPPLE-PEAR CHIFFON PIE*

Prepare pudding as directed. Pour into an 8-inch, prepared pastry shell and chill. Garnish with whipped topping and mint sprigs just before serving.

Yield: 6 servings

LIME CREAM PIE

This deceptively light-tasting pie has over sixteen grams of protein per serving, which makes it an ideal conclusion for a summer salad luncheon or a winter bowl of soup. Smooth, rich and creamy, yet refreshingly tart, half-cup servings as a pudding provide a delightful finish for a vegetarian meal. However it is served, the beneficial bioflavonoids from the whole limes are present.

1½ tablespoons PURE GELATIN
¾ cup water, divided
2 large limes (200 grams)
½ cup plus 1 tablespoon TUR-BINADO SUGAR (divided)
⅓ cup non-instant SKIM MILK POWDER
¼ cup FRUCTOSE GRANULES
¼ teaspoon C-TRATE

1½ cups low-fat cottage cheese (recipe for homemade cottage cheese on page 52)
2 ice cubes
1 large egg white
¼ teaspoon pure vanilla
¼ cup GROUND COCONUT
1 baked Wheat Pastry shell (recipe on page 223)

Sprinkle gelatin on ½ cup of the water and let stand for 5 minutes. Heat and stir in a small saucepan until gelatin is dissolved. (Or microwave on full power for 1 minute in a glass measuring cup.) Pour gelatin mixture into the container of an electric blender.

Grate 1 teaspoon lime peel and add to the blender. Peel limes, quarter and remove any seeds. Add to blender with ½ cup sugar, skim milk powder, fructose, C-Trate and the remaining quarter cup water. Blend on high speed for 30 seconds. Add cottage cheese and blend until smooth, pushing down the sides as necessary. Add ice cubes one at a time and blend until ice is dissolved. Chill for a few minutes until slightly thickened. Beat egg white until foamy, then beat in the tablespoon of sugar and the vanilla. Fold into lime mixture with the coconut. Pile into the prepared pie shell and refrigerate until serving time.

Yield: 6 servings

MAPLE-NUT PIE

This incredible pie is so mellow and rich-tasting that no one would ever suspect it of being a vitamin-mineral supplement. Serve as a festive finale to a simple luncheon or light supper and the delightful memory will linger long after the nutrients have served their purpose.

⅓ cup non-instant SKIM MILK POWDER
1 tablespoon PURE GELATIN
¼ teaspoon SEA SALT
¼ teaspoon ground cinnamon
½ cup chopped pecans
1¼ pounds carrots, peeled or scraped
¾ cup PURE MAPLE SYRUP, divided
⅔ cup water
2 large eggs, separated

1 teaspoon BLACKSTRAP MOLASSES
½ cup heavy whipping cream
¼ teaspoon pure maple flavoring (optional)
1 baked, 9-inch Wheat Pastry shell (recipe on page 223)
Optional Garnish: Whipped topping or additional whipped cream, sweetened with maple syrup, if desired
Pecan halves

Combine skim milk powder, gelatin, salt, cinnamon and pecans in a saucepan.

Cut carrots in chunks and liquefy one-third at a time in an electric blender, using ½ cup of the maple syrup as the liquid with the first batch. Stir into the dry ingredients in the saucepan. Blend the remaining carrots with ⅓ cup of the water and 1 egg yolk for each third of the carrots. Stir into the mixture in the saucepan with the molasses. (Be sure to remove any tell-tale carrot chunks that might have been lurking beneath the blender blades!) Cook and stir over low heat for about 25 minutes—the mixture should come to a boil to avoid any hint of raw carrot flavor. Cover and let stand to cool, or chill in a bowl of ice cubes and water.

Beat the egg whites until frothy. Heat the remaining one-fourth cup syrup to boiling in a small pan. Continue beating the egg whites while slowly adding the boiling syrup. Beat until stiff and glossy. Whip cream and fold into the egg whites. Fold mixture into the cooled filling. Taste and add the maple flavoring, if desired. Pile into pastry shell and chill for several hours. Garnish with whipped topping and pecan halves just before serving.

TO MICROWAVE: Prepare filling as for conventional cooking, but use a 2-quart cooking dish. Cover and microwave on full power for 5 minutes. Stir, leave uncovered and microwave on full power for 10 minutes, stirring each 2 or 3 minutes. Cool and combine with remaining ingredients as directed, heating the ¼-cup syrup in a glass measuring cup for 1 minute before drizzling it into the egg whites.

SUPER-NUTRITION VARIATION:

● Add with the molasses before cooking:
  1 tablespoon LIQUID LECITHIN
  ¼ teaspoon C-TRATE
  contents of 1 DAILY B-COMPLEX capsule

Yield: 6 servings

BARTLETT PIE TART

Bigger than a tart, better than a pie, this combination of fresh pears with a crumbly rich, whole grain crust makes a memorable dessert with a full complement of vitamins and minerals, plus fiber and protein.

Crust:

½ cup unsifted UNBLEACHED WHITE FLOUR
½ cup GRAHAM FLOUR
2 tablespoons WHEAT GERM
¼ teaspoon SEA SALT

6 tablespoons safflower margarine
1 egg yolk
1 tablespoon RAW HONEY
1 teaspoon lemon juice

Filling:

2 large, fresh Bartlett pears (or 2 cups chopped, sugar-free, canned pears)
2 tablespoons ARROWROOT or cornstarch, divided
¼ cup RAW BROWN SUGAR

¼ teaspoon SEA SALT
¼ teaspoon ground cinnamon
6 tablespoons water
1 tablespoon safflower margarine
1 teaspoon lemon juice
½ teaspoon pure vanilla

Make the crust by first combining the flours, wheat germ and salt in a mixing bowl or food processor. Cut in margarine, then mix in egg yolk, honey and lemon juice until moist but crumbly. Reserve ⅓ cup for topping and press the remainder into the bottom and 1 inch up the sides of an oiled 9 × 5-inch loaf pan. Bake for 10 minutes in a preheated, 375 degree oven.

While the crust is baking, wash pears, remove any blemishes, quarter, core and chop into half-inch pieces. (The peelings may be removed if desired, but they provide a lot of fiber when left on the pears.) Toss them with 1 tablespoon of the arrowroot and let stand while making the sauce.

In a small saucepan combine the brown sugar, remaining tablespoon of arrowroot, salt and cinnamon. Gradually blend in the water. Cook and stir over medium heat until thickened. Stir in the tablespoon of margarine, teaspoon of lemon juice and the vanilla.

Spread the chopped pears in the partially baked shell, cover with sauce and crumble the reserved crust dough over the top. Bake for 25 to 30 minutes at 375 degrees, removing before the sides become browned.

TO MICROWAVE: Make crust as directed. Press into a glass pan and microwave on full power for 3 minutes, rotating one-half turn after 2 minutes. (Elevating the pan on a rack will allow the microwaves to better penetrate the center.)

Toss the chopped pears with 1 tablespoon of arrowroot in a 4-cup glass measure and let stand. Combine brown sugar, remaining tablespoon of arrowroot, salt and cinnamon in a 2-cup glass measure. Microwave on full power for 2 minutes, stirring once. Stir in margarine, lemon juice and vanilla. Gently stir the hot sauce into the pears and microwave for 3 minutes on full power, stirring once. Spread the simmering mixture in the partially baked shell and crumble the reserved crust dough over the top. Place on a rack and microwave for 2 minutes on full power. Rotate one-half turn, set the control on Defrost (half power) and microwave for 2 more minutes.

The pie-tart freezes beautifully, defrosts quickly if cut into individual servings before freezing, and may be served either warm or cold.

SUPER-NUTRITION VARIATION:

- Combine with the dry ingredients for the crust:
  2 tablespoons LECITHIN GRANULES
  ½ teaspoon DOLOMITE POWDER
  ¼ teaspoon B-COMPLEX POWDER
- Stir ¼ teaspoon C-TRATE into the sauce with the vanilla

Yield: 4 generous servings

For a more elaborate presentation: bake the pie-tart in an 8-inch round baking dish or pie plate, cut into six servings and accompany each one with a wedge of mellow cheddar cheese or a scoop of homemade ice cream.

GREEN TOMATO PIE

Call this a "mystery pie" and let your diners guess that the filling is apricot, apple or plum before revealing the real ingredients!

½ cup RAW BROWN SUGAR
¼ cup FRUCTOSE GRANULES
¼ cup STONE-GROUND WHOLE WHEAT FLOUR
½ teaspoon ground cinnamon
½ teaspoon SEA SALT
¼ teaspoon ground nutmeg
3 tablespoons water
1 teaspoon grated lemon peel

3½ cups chopped green tomatoes (1¼ pounds)
2 tablespoons safflower margarine
2 tablespoons LECITHIN GRANULES
¼ teaspoon C-TRATE
1 recipe Wheat Pastry (recipe on page 223)

In a 2-quart saucepan, combine brown sugar, fructose, flour, cinnamon, salt and nutmeg. Blend in water and lemon peel, stirring until smooth. Wash tomatoes, remove cores and blemishes but do not peel unless tomatoes are beginning to ripen and the skins are tough. Chop by hand or in a food processor and stir into the sugar mixture. Cook and stir over medium heat until thickened and boiling. Stir in margarine, lecithin granules and C-Trate and let stand for 10 minutes.

Prepare pastry and divide, allowing slightly more than half for the bottom crust. Pour filling into pastry-lined, 9-inch pie plate, moisten edges with water and cover with top crust. Press edges to seal and flute or score with the tines of a fork. Make small slashes in a decorative pattern in the top crust to allow the steam to escape. Place on a baking sheet to catch any drippings and bake in a preheated 400 degree oven for 40 minutes.

TO MICROWAVE: In a 1½-quart cooking dish, combine brown sugar, fructose, flour, cinnamon, salt and nutmeg. Blend in water and lemon peel, stirring until smooth. Stir in chopped tomatoes and microwave, uncovered, on full power until thickened and boiling—about 8 minutes—stirring each 2 minutes. Stir in margarine, lecithin granules and C-Trate and let stand for 10 minutes.

Prepare pastry and divide, allowing slightly more than one half for the bottom crust. Pour filling into pastry-lined 9-inch glass pie plate, moisten edges with water and cover with top crust. Press edges to seal and flute or score with the tines of a fork. Make small slashes in a decorative pattern in the top crust to allow the steam to escape. Place on a rack, or an inverted glass pie plate, and microwave for 4 minutes on full power, rotating one-quarter turn after 2 minutes. Turn pie another quarter-turn, set control on half power (or Defrost) and microwave for 4 minutes. Transfer to a preheated 400 degree conventional oven to brown for 15 minutes, or microwave and brown with a micro-wave browning unit according to the manufacturer's directions. Cool before serving with a wedge of cheese or a scoop of homemade ice cream.

Yield: 6 servings

APPLE MERINGUE PIE

A superb apple pie that requires neither cheese nor ice cream as an accompaniment, yet is so filled with nourishment (including almost 10 grams of protein per serving) that one piece can serve as a complete snack or mini-meal.

½ recipe for Wheat Pastry (page 223)
½ cup RAW BROWN SUGAR, firmly packed and divided
⅓ cup TURBINADO SUGAR
⅓ cup non-instant SKIM MILK POWDER
3 tablespoons UNBLEACHED WHITE FLOUR
2 tablespoons SOY FLOUR

½ teaspoon ground cinnamon
¼ teaspoon ground nutmeg
¼ teaspoon SEA SALT
¼ teaspoon C-TRATE
1 5,000 IU SUPER DRY A & D capsule (optional)
1 cup natural APPLE JUICE
3 large eggs, separated
1 tablespoon safflower margarine
¾ teaspoon pure vanilla, divided

1 pound cooking apples, peeled,	⅛ teaspoon SEA SALT
cored and sliced (3 cups)	⅛ teaspoon ground allspice
⅛ teaspoon cream of tartar	

Roll pastry between sheets of waxed paper and line a 9-inch pie pan. Flute the rim but do not prick. Set aside.

Reserve 3 tablespoons of the brown sugar for the meringue and place the remainder in a 2-quart saucepan. Add turbinado sugar, skim milk powder, white and soy flours, cinnamon, nutmeg, ¼ teaspoon salt, C-Trate and the contents of the A and D capsule (if used). Stir to combine, then whisk in the apple juice and egg yolks. Cook over low heat, stirring frequently, until thickened. Stir in margarine, ½ teaspoon vanilla and sliced apples. Turn into the prepared pastry shell and smooth top. Bake in a preheated 375 degree oven for 45 minutes.

Add cream of tartar and ⅛ teaspoon salt to egg whites and beat until frothy. Continue beating while gradually adding reserved brown sugar. When thick and shiny, add allspice and the remaining ¼ teaspoon vanilla.

Lower oven heat to 325 degrees. Pile meringue on the hot pie, swirling into peaks and sealing to the edges. Return to the oven and bake for 20 minutes.

> **TO MICROWAVE:** Roll pastry between sheets of waxed paper and line a 9-inch glass pie plate. Flute the rim and prick the crust with a fork. Microwave on a rack or inverted baking dish for 4½ minutes on full power, rotating one-quarter turn each minute. Set aside.
>
> Stir C-Trate into apples in a 4-cup glass measure, cover and microwave for 8 minutes on full power, stirring once. Let stand, covered.
>
> Reserve 3 tablespoons of the brown sugar for the meringue and place the remainder in a 1½-quart cooking dish. Add turbinado sugar, skim milk powder, white and soy flours, cinnamon, nutmeg, ¼ teaspoon

salt, and the contents of the A and D capsule (if used). Stir to combine, then whisk in the apple juice and egg yolks. Microwave, uncovered, for 5 minutes on full power, stirring once each minute. (Mixture should thicken but not fully boil.) Stir in margarine, ½ teaspoon vanilla and sliced apples. Pour into baked pastry shell and smooth top.

Add cream of tartar and ⅛ teaspoon salt to egg whites and beat until frothy. Continue beating while gradually adding reserved brown sugar. When thick and shiny, add allspice and the remaining ¼ teaspoon vanilla.

Pile on the warm pie filling and swirl meringue to seal to the crust. Microwave on full power for 2½ minutes, turning once. (The brown sugar and spice gives this meringue an appetizing glow of color without browning. If actual browning is preferred, use a microwave browning unit or slide the pie under a conventional broiler for a minute or so.)

Equally delicious when served while still slightly warm or after chilling.

Yield: 6 servings

Emergency Ration

APPLE-LAYER DATE CAKE

This self-layered cake can be either dessert or an emergency ration. The cake will keep in the refrigerator for over a week—or slices may be quick-frozen, then individually wrapped in freezer plastic. Each small slice is packed with vitamins and minerals, and contains as much protein as one egg.

¾ cup DATE SUGAR, divided
½ cup unsifted UNBLEACHED WHITE FLOUR
½ cup WHOLE WHEAT PASTRY FLOUR, not stirred

¼ cup raw WHEAT GERM
¼ cup non-instant SKIM MILK POWDER
contents of 1 10,000 IU SUPER DRY A & D capsule

2 tablespoons SOY FLOUR
2 tablespoons BREWER'S YEAST
1 teaspoon double-acting baking powder
½ teaspoon DOLOMITE POWDER
¼ teaspoon *each* cinnamon and nutmeg
¼ teaspoon SEA SALT
⅛ teaspoon baking soda
1 large, ripe banana cut in 1-inch pieces

½ cup fresh orange juice
2 large eggs, separated
2 tablespoons NATURAL PEANUT BUTTER
1 tablespoon COLD SESAME OIL
1 tablespoon LIQUID LECITHIN
¾ cup chopped walnuts, divided
½ teaspoon pure vanilla
2 large apples (6 ounces each)
Date Topping (recipe follows)

WITH ELECTRIC BLENDER AND CONVENTIONAL OVEN: In large mixing bowl, place ½ cup of the date sugar, white flour, whole wheat pastry flour, wheat germ, skim milk powder, contents of vitamin A and D capsule, soy flour, brewer's yeast, baking powder, dolomite, cinnamon, nutmeg, salt and soda. Stir well to mix. In blender container, combine banana, orange juice, egg yolks, peanut butter, sesame oil and liquid lecithin. Blend on high speed until smooth. Pour into dry ingredients and mix thoroughly. Beat egg whites and fold in with ½ cup of the nuts and the vanilla. Pour half the batter into a greased bundt or angel-food tube pan. Peel apples, if desired; core and thinly slice. Arrange over batter and sprinkle with remainder of date sugar and nuts. Cover with remaining batter. Bake in preheated 350 degree oven until done, about 1 hour. Turn out on serving plate and cover with Date Topping.

WITH FOOD PROCESSOR AND MICROWAVE OVEN: Place cutting blade in processor work bowl and preload with ½ cup of the date sugar, flours, wheat germ, skim milk powder, contents of the vitamin A & D capsule, brewer's yeast, baking powder, dolomite, cinnamon, nutmeg, salt and soda. Process 5 seconds to blend. Add banana, egg yolks, peanut butter, sesame oil and lecithin and process 15 seconds. Scrape down sides, then add orange juice through the feed tube with the processor running. Beat egg whites and stir in with ½ cup of nuts and vanilla, processing 2 on/off turns or pulsations to complete the blending. Spoon half the batter into an oiled microwave baking ring. Peel apples, if desired; core and slice very thin. Arrange over batter. Sprinkle with remaining date sugar and walnuts. Cover with remaining batter. Microwave on full power for 10 minutes, rotating dish one-quarter turn each 2 minutes. Test with wooden pick to be sure cake is done. Let stand 2 minutes and turn out on serving plate. Cover with Date Topping.

NOTE: If you prefer to use your energy in place of electricity—combine dry ingredients in a mixing bowl. Mash banana and stir in egg yolks, peanut butter, sesame oil and liquid lecithin. Add orange juice and mix until thoroughly blended. Stir into dry ingredients. Beat egg whites with a rotary beater and fold in with ½ cup walnuts and the vanilla. Assemble and bake in either a microwave or conventional oven as directed.

DATE TOPPING

¼ cup DATE SUGAR	1 teaspoon NATURAL PEANUT BUTTER
2 tablespoons non-instant SKIM MILK POWDER	2 tablespoons safflower margarine
⅛ teaspoon cinnamon	
pinch SEA SALT	⅛ teaspoon pure vanilla
¼ cup fresh orange juice	⅛ teaspoon C-TRATE

Mix date sugar, skim milk powder, cinnamon and salt in a small saucepan. Stir in orange juice and peanut butter. Cook and stir over low heat until boiling. Stir in margarine, vanilla and vitamin C powder. Spread over top and sides of cake.

TO MICROWAVE: Mix date sugar, dry milk, cinnamon and salt in a 2-cup glass measure. Stir in orange juice and peanut butter and microwave, uncovered, for 1½ minutes on full power—stirring halfway through the cooking. Stir in margarine, vanilla and C-Trate. Spread over top and sides of cake.

NOTE: this topping remains soft and makes a delicious spread for toast.

Yield: 16 servings of cake with topping

CARAMEL SPICE CAKE
(carrot-oats)

An easily prepared, moist and tender spice cake that is so filled with vitamins and minerals it needs no further supplementing.

1 large carrot
1 cup water
⅔ cup ROLLED OATS
3 tablespoons COLD PRESSED SAFFLOWER OIL
2 tablespoons safflower margarine
¾ cup RAW BROWN SUGAR, firmly packed
¼ cup RAW HONEY
½ cup unsifted UNBLEACHED WHITE FLOUR
½ cup WHOLE WHEAT PASTRY FLOUR

⅓ cup non-instant SKIM MILK POWDER
2 tablespoons LECITHIN GRANULES
½ teaspoon double-acting baking powder
¼ teaspoon baking soda
¼ teaspoon SEA SALT
¼ teaspoon *each* ground cinnamon and mace
⅛ teaspoon ground allspice
1 large egg
Caramel Topping (recipe follows)

Peel or scrape carrot, cut in chunks and liquefy in an electric blender with the cup of water. Pour into a 2-quart saucepan and stir in the oats. Cook over medium heat until boiling, stir and let boil for 1 minute. (Or microwave in a 2-quart mixing bowl for 5 minutes on full power.) Cover and let stand for 5 minutes. Stir in oil, margarine, brown sugar and honey.

Combine flours, skim milk powder, lecithin, baking powder, soda, salt and spices. Add to oat mixture and stir in with the egg. Pour into a $6 \times 10 \times 2$-inch baking pan greased with vegetable shortening. Bake in a preheated 350 degree oven about 45 minutes, or until the center springs back when lightly pressed with a fingertip.

TO MICROWAVE: Prepare as directed and pour into an oiled $6 \times 10 \times 2$-inch baking dish. Elevate on a rack or inverted baking dish and microwave for 7 minutes on full power, rotating one-quarter turn each 2 minutes. (The center of the cake should be raised even with the edges and no longer sticky.)

Caramel Topping

½ cup RAW BROWN SUGAR, firmly packed	3 tablespoons safflower margarine, cut in pieces
1 tablespoon non-instant SKIM MILK POWDER	1 tablespoon water
⅛ teaspoon SEA SALT	1 tablespoon WHEAT GERM OIL
½ cup COCONUT MEAL	¼ teaspoon pure vanilla
½ cup chopped walnuts	

Combine sugar, skim milk powder and salt in a small saucepan. Stir in coconut, nuts, margarine and water. Cook and stir over low heat until sugar has melted and mixture is boiling. (Or mix in a 4-cup glass measure and microwave, uncovered, for 4 minutes on full power—stirring after 2 minutes.) Stir in oil and vanilla and spread atop the still-warm cake in the baking container.

Yield: 10 servings

BROWN VELVET CAKE

Intensify the pleasure for chocolate lovers by sprinkling carob chips over the coconut-and-frosting filling for a layer cake—and just don't mention the beets, carob, or other nutritional benefits.

¾ cup unsifted UNBLEACHED WHITE FLOUR	½ cup STONE-GROUND WHOLE WHEAT FLOUR

¼ cup non-instant SKIM MILK POWDER

2 tablespoons CAROB POWDER

1 teaspoon double-acting baking powder

½ teaspoon SEA SALT

½ cup firmly packed RAW BROWN SUGAR

¼ cup safflower margarine at room temperature

2 tablespoons FRUCTOSE GRANULES

1 large egg plus 2 large egg whites

¾ cup water, divided

1 large raw beet, scrubbed and trimmed but not peeled (100 grams)

1 tablespoon APPLE CIDER VINEGAR

¾ teaspoon pure vanilla

½ teaspoon baking soda

Combine flours, skim milk powder, carob, baking powder and salt and set aside. Place brown sugar, margarine, fructose and the whole egg in the small bowl of an electric mixer. Beat for 3 minutes on medium speed, or beat by hand until fluffy.

Cut beet in chunks and liquefy with ½ cup of the water in an electric blender. Add to the sugar mixture. Rinse blender with remaining water and stir in vinegar, vanilla and soda. Add to the mixer bowl with dry ingredients. Beat on medium speed for 2 minutes, or by hand until creamy smooth. Beat egg whites until stiff and fold into the batter.

Pour into a 6 × 10 × 2-inch baking pan or dish greased with vegetable shortening. Bake in a preheated 350 degree oven for 45 to 50 minutes—until a toothpick inserted in the center comes out clean.

TO MICROWAVE: Reduce baking powder to ¾ teaspoon and baking soda to ¼ teaspoon. Prepare cake batter as directed and pour into an oiled 6 × 10 × 2-inch baking dish. Microwave on a rack or an inverted baking dish for 9 minutes on full power, rotating dish one-quarter turn each 2 minutes. (Cake is done when a wooden toothpick inserted in the center comes out clean even though the surface may still be moist.)

Frost cake in the cooking container and cut in squares to serve. If desired, turn out on a rack to cool and cut in half to make a layer cake. Fill with ½ cup Marshmallow

Frosting (recipe on page 246) mixed with ¼ cup GROUND COCONUT and/or CAROB CHIPS. Swirl the remaining frosting over the top and sides of the cake.

SUPER-NUTRITION VARIATION:

- Combine with the dry ingredients:
  ¼ teaspoon DOLOMITE POWDER
  contents of 1 DAILY B COMPLEX capsule
  contents of 1 5000 IU SUPER DRY A & D capsule
  ⅛ teaspoon C-TRATE
- Add 1 tablespoon LIQUID LECITHIN with the margarine

Yield: 8 servings

SEED CAKES

Seed cakes, glazed and thinly sliced, were a tea-time favorite in colonial days. Modern appliances take the work out of preparation; wheat germ, lecithin and alfalfa or chia seeds add nutrients; and what isn't daintily nibbled from the tea tray or for dessert may be spread with butter and munched for a delightful snack.

POPPY-SEED CAKE

2 tablespoons poppy seeds
2 tablespoons CHIA SEEDS
⅓ cup water
½ cup TURBINADO SUGAR
¼ cup safflower margarine at room temperature
2 large eggs
2 tablespoons LIQUID LECITHIN
2 tablespoons RAW HONEY

½ teaspoon pure vanilla
1 cup unsifted UNBLEACHED WHITE FLOUR
¼ cup non-instant SKIM MILK POWDER
2 tablespoons WHEAT GERM
1 teaspoon double acting baking powder
¼ teaspoon SEA SALT

Combine seeds with water and let stand, covered, for 4 to 12 hours.

In a small mixing bowl, combine the seeds with the sugar, margarine, eggs, lecithin, honey and vanilla. Beat on medium speed for 1 minute, or by hand until creamy.

Combine the flour, skim milk powder, wheat germ, baking powder and salt. Stir into the seed mixture and beat by hand or on medium speed with an electric mixer for 2 minutes.

Pour into a loaf pan that has been greased with vegetable shortening and bottom-lined with a strip of parchment paper. Bake in a preheated 350 degree oven for about 1 hour, or until a toothpick inserted in the center comes out clean. Turn out on a rack, remove parchment paper and immediately invert onto the serving plate so the cake is right-side up.

> **TO MICROWAVE:** Prepare cake as directed but pour into a glass loaf pan that has been oiled and bottom-lined with parchment paper. Let stand for 5 minutes. Microwave on a rack or inverted baking dish for 6½ minutes—or until a toothpick inserted in the center comes out clean—turning each 2 minutes. Invert onto serving plate and remove parchment paper. (Leave upside-down to conceal any irregularities in the raised top of the cake.)

BROWN SUGAR GLAZE

⅓ cup RAW BROWN SUGAR, firmly packed
1 tablespoon non-instant SKIM MILK POWDER
⅛ teaspoon SEA SALT
1½ tablespoons water
1 teaspoon safflower margarine
¼ teaspoon pure vanilla
⅛ teaspoon C-TRATE

Combine sugar, skim milk powder and sea salt in a small skillet or saucepan. Stir in water and cook over low heat until fully boiling—stirring constantly. (Or combine sugar, dry milk, salt and water in a 2-cup glass measure and microwave on full power for 1½ minutes, stirring after 1 minute.) Stir in margarine, vanilla and C-Trate. Spread over the top of the cake, allowing rivulets to trickle down the sides and ends.

VARIATION: *CARAWAY SEED CAKE:*

- Substitute 2 tablespoons CARAWAY SEED for the poppy seed

- Substitute 2 tablespoons ALFALFA SEED for the chia seed

Yield: 18 standard slices

LOW-CARBOHYDRATE ANGEL FOOD CAKE

Always a dieter's delight with no fat, little flour, and lots of protein; fructose and Substi-Sweet makes this Angel Food even more appealing. Arrowroot sifted with the dry ingredients gives unbleached white flour the lightness of highly refined cake flour.

½ cup unsifted UNBLEACHED
   WHITE FLOUR
1½ tablespoons FRUCTOSE
   GRANULES
1½ teaspoons ARROWROOT or
   cornstarch
¼ teaspoon SEA SALT
¼ teaspoon C-TRATE

6 large egg whites
2 teaspoons water
½ teaspoon cream of tartar
1½ teaspoons liquid SUBSTI-
   SWEET
¼ teaspoon almond flavoring
¼ teaspoon pure vanilla

Combine flour, fructose, arrowroot, salt and vitamin C powder and sift together three times. Set aside.

Beat egg whites with water until frothy. Add cream of tartar and beat until stiff. Beat in Substi-Sweet, almond and vanilla flavorings. Sift in dry ingredients and fold to combine.

Spoon into an ungreased tube or loaf pan and bake in a preheated, 350 degree oven for 25 to 30 minutes—until a toothpick inserted in the center comes out clean. Invert pan on a rack to cool before removing cake.

TO MICROWAVE: *Theoretically, Angel Food cakes cannot be microwaved, but this recipe hasn't been informed of this fact, so it microwaves beautifully—just don't over-bake or it will toughen.*

Prepare as directed and spoon into a microwave baking ring. Place on a rack or an inverted baking dish and microwave on full power for 3½ to 4 minutes—until cake pulls away from the outside of the dish. Let stand 2 minutes and turn out onto serving plate.

SUPER-NUTRITION VARIATION:

For those who need a little extra calcium, sift with the flour: ¼ teaspoon DOLOMITE POWDER
¼ teaspoon BONE MEAL POWDER

Yield: 8 servings

GLORIFIED ANGEL DESSERT

For a heavenly dessert to be enjoyed with a clear conscience:

Cube half the Angel Food cake with 2 forks or a cakebreaker and combine with 1½ cups fresh peaches or strawberries and either of the Whipped Toppings from pages 247-248.

Yield: 4 generous servings

HONEY-WHITE CAKE

Cholesterol-free and neither powdery-light nor squishy-soft, this sturdy little white cake with a delicate flavor holds its own with all types of fillings and frostings.

1 cup plus 2 tablespoons unsifted UNBLEACHED WHITE FLOUR	½ teaspoon SEA SALT
3 tablespoons non-instant SKIM MILK POWDER	2 large egg whites
1 tablespoon ARROWROOT or cornstarch	⅛ teaspoon cream of tartar
1¼ teaspoons double acting baking powder	½ cup TURBINADO SUGAR
	⅔ cup water
	3 tablespoons RAW HONEY
	6 tablespoons COLD PRESSED ALMOND OIL

Preheat oven to 350 degrees for glass pans, 375 degrees if using metal. To serve right from the pan, use an 8 × 8 × 2-inch pan greased with vegetable shortening; to make a layer cake, grease a $7 \times 11 \times 2$-inch pan and line the bottom with parchment or waxed paper.

Combine the flour, skim milk powder, arrowroot, baking powder and salt. Sift into a large mixing bowl and set aside.

Place the egg whites and cream of tartar in a small mixing bowl and beat until frothy. Continue beating while gradually adding sugar and beat until thick and glossy. Set aside.

Mix honey with water and stir into the dry ingredients with the oil. Beat on low speed for 3 minutes with an electric mixer, or by hand until creamy-smooth. Fold in beaten egg whites. Pour into prepared pan and bake for approximately 30 minutes—until a toothpick inserted in the center comes out clean.

Cool the square cake in its pan on a rack and frost as desired. For a layer cake, turn out the rectangular cake, remove waxed paper and let cool. Cut in half, crosswise, fill and frost as desired.

TO MICROWAVE: Reduce baking powder to 1 teaspoon and mix the cake as directed. Using smaller pans assures even microwave baking and two shallow, square, one-quart casseroles are ideal for this cake. (If you don't have two matching casseroles, one casserole can be washed between bakings and used for both halves of the batter.) Oil the baking dish and bottom-line with waxed or parchment paper. Pour in half the batter and place on a rack or an inverted baking dish in the microwave oven. Microwave on full power for 4 minutes, rotating dish one-quarter turn each minute. (Cake should be pulling away from the sides of the dish and a toothpick inserted in the center should come out clean.) Turn out on a sheet of waxed paper over a metal cake rack. Wash the baking dish (if necessary), oil, line and repeat with the second half of the batter. Frost and cut in squares to serve, or split the two cakes to make four thin layers and put together with a filling before frosting.

For a spectacularly nutritious LADY BALTIMORE CAKE, spread Fruit and Nut Filling between the layers and frost sides and top with Honey Fluff frosting (recipe on page 246).

Yield: 8 servings

FRUIT & NUT CAKE FILLING

⅓ cup firmly packed RAW BROWN SUGAR
⅓ cup non-instant SKIM MILK POWDER
2 tablespoons ARROWROOT or cornstarch
⅛ teaspoon SEA SALT
⅔ cup water
¼ cup ORANGE BLOSSOM HONEY

½ cup chopped walnuts
¼ cup chopped CALIMYRNA FIGS
¼ cup chopped CALIFORNIA DATES
1 teaspoon grated orange peel
¼ cup COCONUT MEAL
⅛ teaspoon C-TRATE

In a small, heavy-bottomed saucepan, mix brown sugar, skim milk powder, arrowroot and salt. Gradually stir in water. Add honey and stir over low heat until sugar is dissolved. Add nuts, figs, dates and orange peel.

Cook until thickened and bubbling, stirring frequently. Stir in coconut meal and C-Trate.

TO MICROWAVE: Combine brown sugar, skim milk powder, arrowroot and salt in a 4-cup glass measure. Gradually stir in water and honey. Microwave on full power for 1 minute. Stir in nuts, figs, dates and orange peel. Microwave, uncovered, on full power until thickened and bubbling—about 5 minutes—stirring after 2 minutes and then once each minute. Stir in coconut meal and C-Trate.

Let cool before spreading between layers for 1 large or 2 small cakes.

SUPER-NUTRITION VARIATION:

- Stir in with the coconut meal: 2 tablespoons LECITHIN GRANULES.
  contents of 1 10,000 IU SUPER DRY A & D capsule
  contents of 1 DAILY B COMPLEX capsule

Yield: 1½ cups

HONEY FLUFF FROSTING

Easy to prepare, delightful to spread, beautiful to look at and delicious to eat, this fat-free frosting contains nothing but the natural nutrients of honey (or maple syrup) and egg whites.

2 large egg whites	**1 cup RAW HONEY**
⅛ teaspoon SEA SALT	**⅛ teaspoon C-TRATE**

Place egg whites and salt in the small bowl of an electric mixer and beat until stiff. Heat honey to boiling in a small saucepan on the stove or in a 2-cup glass measure in the microwave oven—allowing 3 minutes of microwaving on full power. Continue beating the egg whites while gradually adding the honey. Add the C-Trate. Beat for another minute or so, until the frosting is very thick and shiny. Swirl on the sides and top of one large or two small layer cakes.

VARIATION: *MAPLE FLUFF FROSTING:*

- Substitute 1 cup PURE MAPLE SYRUP for the honey and proceed as directed

Yield: 16 servings

MARSHMALLOW FROSTING

Quicker and easier than a "Seven-minute Frosting," because your stand mixer will do all the work without the bother of holding a beater in the top of a double-boiler. (To make this with a rotary beater you'll need a kitchen-helper or a third hand.) The small amount of gelatin gives body to the frosting with less than half the usual amount of sugar.

1 large egg white	2 tablespoons water
⅛ teaspoon cream of tartar	2 tablespoons RAW HONEY
3 tablespoons TURBINADO SUGAR	¼ teaspoon pure vanilla
¾ teaspoon PURE GELATIN	⅛ teaspoon C-TRATE

Beat egg white and cream of tartar until frothy in the small bowl of an electric mixer. Combine sugar, gelatin, water and honey in a small saucepan and heat to boiling. (Or combine in a 1-cup glass measure and microwave for 1 minute.) Continue beating egg whites on the highest speed while slowly drizzling in the hot liquid. Continue beating until frosting is very thick and shiny. Beat in vanilla and C-Trate.

Makes enough filling and frosting for the 8-serving Brown Velvet or Honey-White layer cakes. For larger layer cakes, the recipe may be doubled.

WHIPPED TOPPINGS

Two solutions for avoiding the calories and fat in heavy cream and the additives in commercial imitations, and still indulge in "whipped cream." The skim milk powder in Topping #1 offers additional protein and calcium when there is time for advance preparation—while the banana-egg white Topping #2 can come to the rescue for quick-fix treats.

WHIPPED TOPPING #1—SKIM MILK POWDER

½ teaspoon PURE GELATIN	½ cup non-instant SKIM MILK POWDER
1 teaspoon FRUCTOSE GRANULES	3 ice cubes
⅓ cup water	½ teaspoon pure vanilla
	¼ teaspoon C-TRATE

Combine gelatin and fructose in a small saucepan. Stir in water and heat to simmering. (Or combine in a 1-cup glass measure and microwave for 45 seconds.) Pour into the

container of an electric blender. Add skim milk powder
and blend for 5 seconds. Scrape down sides and blend on
high speed while adding ice cubes one at a time. Add
vanilla and C-Trate and blend until ice is melted. Pour into
the small bowl of an electric mixer and freeze until ice
crystals form around the edge. Beat with the mixer on high
speed until very thick. (This whipped cream won't turn to
butter!) Serve immediately or refrigerate for several hours
in a covered container.

Yield: 13 servings of 3 tablespoons each

WHIPPED TOPPING #2—BANANA

1 large egg white	½ teaspoon pure vanilla
½ large banana (100 grams)	⅛ teaspoon C-TRATE

Beat egg white in the small bowl of an electric mixer until
fluffy. Gradually add thinly sliced banana and continue
beating on high speed until thick. Lift beaters and scrape
down the sides of the bowl to incorporate any flecks of
banana. Add vanilla and C-Trate, then beat until very
thick. Serve at once.

Yield: 6 servings of 3 tablespoons each

Emergency Ration

"CHOCOLATE CHIP" COOKIES

*The world's greatest survival ration—utterly delicious chocolate
chip cookies! Just don't mention carob or brewer's yeast and no
one will dream that what they're eating is good for them! (Note
to weight watchers: Putting nutrition in doesn't take the calories
out.)*

1 cup unsifted UNBLEACHED WHITE FLOUR	½ cup WHOLE WHEAT PASTRY FLOUR

⅔ cup RAW BROWN SUGAR, firmly packed
½ cup ROLLED OATS
1 tablespoon BREWER'S YEAST
1 10,000 IU SUPER DRY A & D capsule
½ teaspoon double-acting baking powder
½ teaspoon DOLOMITE POWDER

¼ teaspoon SEA SALT
½ cup (1 stick) safflower margarine
1 large egg
2 tablespoons LECITHIN GRANULES
1 teaspoon pure vanilla
½ cup CAROB NUGGETS
½ cup chopped PECANS

Place flours, sugar, oats, brewer's yeast, vitamin A and D from the capsule, baking powder, dolomite and salt in a large mixing bowl. Beat on low speed with the mixer (or by hand) to blend. Add margarine and cut in or beat on medium speed. Add egg, lecithin and vanilla. Beat until mixed. Stir in carob and nuts. (Mixture will be crumbly.) Scoop out 2 tablespoons at a time and shape into balls. Flatten to about ¼-inch and place on ungreased baking sheets.

Bake in a preheated, 350 degree oven for about 12 minutes—cookies should not brown. Loosen immediately to prevent sticking.

TO MICROWAVE: Mix cookies as directed. Cut parchment paper into 2-inch strips and place around the outside of a plastic baking sheet. Arrange 9 cookies on the strips and microwave on full power for 3 minutes, turning dish after 2 minutes. Lift cookies to paper towels, turn over parchment strips and microwave the next 9 cookies. (Microwaving all the cookies at once does not save any kitchen time, but is convenient and energy saving when you refrigerate part of the dough and microwave a few at a time, as needed.)

Yield: 3 dozen large cookies

FRUIT & NUT BONBONS

The nostalgic flavor of an old-fashioned confection—updated for modern preparation, taste, and nutrition. Wonderful to serve and to gift wrap at Christmas time, they are also a delight for summer nibbling as neither cooking nor baking is required.

½ cup SUNFLOWER SEEDS
½ cup RAW WHEAT GERM
½ cup NATURALLY DRIED DATES
½ cup NATURALLY DRIED FIGS
½ cup seedless RAISINS
½ cup chopped walnuts

½ cup NATURAL ALMOND, CASHEW or PEANUT BUTTER
¼ teaspoon SEA SALT
1 teaspoon pure vanilla
½ cup CAROB NUGGETS
½ cup COCONUT MEAL

Finely chop sunflower seeds and wheat germ in processor or electric blender. Grind dates, figs, raisins and walnuts with a food grinder or in the processor. (If using a food processor, leave the seed mixture in the processor bowl and add the dates, etc.)

Process or stir in the nut butter, salt and vanilla (with the seeds and wheat germ if they were in the blender), then process or stir in the carob nuggets. Shape by rounded teaspoonfuls into balls and roll in the coconut. Store in a tightly covered container, or freeze for longer storage.

SUPER-NUTRITION VARIATION:

Combine with the chopped sunflower seeds and wheat germ:

- 1 teaspoon DOLOMITE POWDER
- ¼ teaspoon B-COMPLEX POWDER
- ¼ teaspoon C-TRATE
- contents of 1 10,000 IU SUPER DRY A & D capsule

Yield: 4 dozen bonbons

GNC Ingredients

The numbers following the ingredients are for convenience in ordering by mail from General Nutrition Corporation; other items are available in local GNC Health Food Stores.

A & D VITAMINS, SUPER DRY #202

ACIDOPHILUS CULTURE #996

ALFALFA SEEDS #504

ALL BLEND OIL, COLD PRESSED #1494

ALL-STAR 95% PROTEIN SUPREME POWDER #1420

ALMOND BUTTER #505

ALMOND OIL, COLD PRESSED #1490

APPLE CIDER VINEGAR #1350

APPLE JUICE, NATURAL #2901

ARROWROOT FLOUR #495

B-COMPLEX, DAILY CAPSULE WITH VITAMIN C #837

B-COMPLEX YEAST POWDER #673

BLACK-EYED PEAS #1454

BLACKSTRAP MOLASSES #1392

BONE MEAL POWDER #512

BRAN, PURE UNPROCESSED #1354

BREWER'S YEAST POWDER #516, FLAKES #515,
  PRIMARY GROWN #788

BUCKWHEAT FLOUR #492

BULGUR WHEAT #3700

C-TRATE, VITAMIN C POWDER OR CRYSTALS #494

CAROB CANDY BARS #699, 698, 561, 709

CAROB NUGGETS #1244

CAROB POWDER #521

CASHEW BUTTER, NATURAL #522

CHIA SEEDS #568

COCONUT MEAL #351

CORNMEAL, WHOLE GROUND WHITE #469

DATE SUGAR #511

DATES #519

DOLOMITE POWDER #667

FIGS, BLACK MISSION #510

FIGS CALIMYRNA #520

FRUCTOSE POWDER #426

GARBANZOS = CHICK PEAS OR CECI BEANS #1439

GELATIN #563

GLUTEN FLOUR #489

GRAHAM FLOUR #508

HONEY, ORANGE BLOSSOM #741

HONEY, RAW = CLOVER HONEY #743, TUPELO HONEY
#742, or WILD FLOWER HONEY #1252

INSTANT LIQUID TENDERIZER, #1445

KELP, GRANULATED #369

KELP SEASONING #678

LECITHIN GRANULES #s 56 and 96

LENTILS #1436

LIQUID LECITHIN #1390

MAPLE SYRUP PURE #1407

MILLET #572

MILLET, GROUND MEAL #571

OAT FLOUR #277

OATMEAL, ROLLED—(ROLLED OATS) #279

OATMEAL, STEEL CUT #280

OLIVE OIL #1493

PEANUT BUTTER, NATURAL #205

PEANUT OIL, COLD PRESSED #1497

PECANS, HALVES #1433.

PRUNES, LARGE #590

PRUNES, MEDIUM #565

PUMPKIN SEED MEAL #661

PUMPKIN SEEDS #591

RAISINS, THOMPSON #1379

RAISINS, MONUKKA #728

RICE FLOUR #499

RICE, NATURAL BROWN #714

RYE FLOUR #484

SAFFLOWER OIL, COLD PRESSED = SAFFLOWER
  SEED OIL #599

SEA SALT #601

SESAME OIL, COLD PRESSED #1500

SESAME SEEDS #603

SKIM MILK POWDER, NON-INSTANT #487

SOYBEANS, YELLOW #480

SOYBEAN LECITHIN GRANULES #96

SOY FLOUR #483

SOY GRITS #275

SPIKE #581

SUBSTI-SWEET, LIQUID #97

SUNFLOWER SEED MEAL #607

SUNFLOWER SEEDS #608

TAMARI SOY SAUCE #1076

TURBINADO SUGAR #488

UNBLEACHED WHITE FLOUR = UNBLEACHED FLOUR
  #486

VEGE-SAL #600

VEGETABLE SALAD POWDER #654

VITAMIN C POWDER or CRYSTALS = C-TRATE #494

WALNUT OIL, COLD PRESSED #149

WHEAT GERM OIL #45

WHEAT GERM, RAW #648

WHEAT GERM, TOASTED #649

WHEY POWDER #650

WHOLE WHEAT FLOUR #485

YELLOW CORNMEAL #271

Guide to Vitamins & Minerals

A Guide To Vitamins And Minerals

VITAMIN	BEST SOURCES	MAIN ROLES	DEFICIENCY SYMPTOMS
A	Liver; eggs; cheese; butter, fortified margarine and milk; yellow, orange and dark green vegetables (e.g., carrots, broccoli, squash, spinach).	Formation and maintenance of skin and mucous membranes; bone growth; vision; reproduction; teeth.	Night blindness; rough skin and mucous membranes; no bone growth; cracked, decayed teeth; drying of eyes.
Thiamin (B1)	Pork (especially ham); liver, oysters; whole grain and enriched cereals, pasta and bread; wheat germ; brewer's yeast; green peas.	Release of energy from carbohydrates; synthesis of nerve-regulating substance.	Beriberi: mental confusion; muscular weakness; swelling of heart; leg cramps.
Riboflavin (B2)	Liver, milk, meat, dark green vegetables, whole grain and enriched cereals, pasta and bread, mushrooms.	Release of energy to cells from carbohydrates, proteins and fats; maintenance of mucous membranes.	Skin disorders, especially around nose and lips; cracks at mouth corners, eyes very sensitive to light.
Niacin (B3)	Liver; poultry; meat; tuna; whole grain and enriched cereals, pasta and bread; nuts, dried beans and peas. Made in body from amino acid tryptophan.	Works with thiamin and riboflavin in energy-producing reactions in cells.	Pellagra: skin disorders, especially parts exposed to sun; smooth tongue; diarrhea; mental confusion; irritability.
Pyridoxine (B6)	Whole grain (but not enriched) cereals and bread; liver; avocados; spinach; green beans; bananas.	Absorption and metabolism of proteins; use of fats; formation of red blood cells.	Skin disorders: cracks at mouth corners; smooth tongue; convulsions; dizziness; nausea; anemia; kidney stones.
Cobalamin (B12)	Liver; kidneys; meat; fish; eggs; milk; oysters.	Building of genetic material, formation of red blood cells, functioning of nervous system.	Pernicious anemia: anemia; degeneration of peripheral nerves.
Folic acid (Folacin)	Liver; kidneys; dark green leafy vegetables; wheat germ; brewer's yeast.	Assists in forming body proteins and genetic material; formation of hemoglobin.	Anemia with large red blood cells; smooth tongue; diarrhea
Pantothenic acid	Liver; kidneys; whole grain bread and cereal; nuts; eggs; dark green vegetables; yeast.	Metabolism of carbohydrates, proteins and fats; formation of hormones and nerve-regulating substances.	Not known except experimentally in man: vomiting, abdominal pain; fatigue; sleep problems.

261

VITAMIN	BEST SOURCES	MAIN ROLES	DEFICIENCY SYMPTOMS
Biotin	Egg yolk: liver: kidneys: dark green vegetables: green beans. Made in intestinal tract.	Formation of fatty acids: release of energy from carbohydrates.	Not known except experimentally in man: fatigue: depression: nausea: pains: loss of appetite.
C (Ascorbic acid)	Many fruits and vegetables, including citrus, tomato, strawberries, melon, green pepper, potato, dark green vegetables.	Maintenance of health of bones, teeth, blood vessels: formation of collagen, which supports body structure; anti-oxidant.	Scurvy: gums bleed: muscles degenerate: wounds don't heal: skin rough, brown and dry: teeth loosen.
D	Milk: egg yolk: liver: tuna: salmon. Made on skin in sunlight.	Essential for normal bone growth and maintenance of strong bones.	Rickets (in children): retarded growth: bowed legs: malformed teeth: protruding abdomen. Osteomalacia (in adults): bones soften, deform and fracture easily: muscular twitching and spasms.
E	Vegetable oils: margarine: whole grain cereal and bread: wheat germ: liver: dried beans: green leafy vegetables.	Formation of red blood cells, muscle and other tissues: prevents oxidation of vitamin A and fats.	Breakdown of red blood cells. Symptoms in animals (reproductive failure, liver degeneration, muscular dystrophy, etc.) not seen in man.
K	Green leafy vegetables: vegetables in cabbage family: milk. Made in intestinal tract.	Essential for normal blood clotting.	Hemorrhage (especially in newborns).
MINERAL			
Calcium	Milk, cheese, molasses, yogurt, bone meal, dolomite, almonds, liver (beef).	Bone/tooth formation, blood clotting, heart rhythm, nerve tranquilization, nerve transmission, muscle growth & contraction.	Heart palpitations, insomnia, muscle cramps, nervousness, arm & leg numbness, tooth decay.
Chromium	Brewer's yeast, clams, corn oil, whole grain cereals.	Blood sugar level, glucose metabolism (energy).	Atherosclerosis, glucose intolerance in diabetics.
Copper	Legumes, nuts, organ meats, seafood, raisins, molasses, bone meal, soy beans.	Bone formation, hair & skin color, healing processes of body, hemoglobin & red blood cell formation.	General weakness, impaired respiration, skin sores.

Mineral	Sources	Functions	Deficiency Symptoms
Iodine	Seafood, kelp tablets, salt (iodized).	Energy production, metabolism (excess fat), physical & mental development.	Cold hands & feet, dry hair, irritability, nervousness, obesity.
Iron	Blackstrap molasses, eggs, fish, organ meats, poultry, wheat germ, desiccated liver, shredded wheat.	Hemoglobin production, stress & disease resistance.	Breathing difficulties, brittle nails, iron deficiency anemia (pale skin, fatigue), constipation.
Magnesium	Bran, honey, green vegetables, nuts, seafood, spinach, bone meal, kelp tablets.	Acid/alkaline balance, blood sugar metabolism (energy), metabolism (calcium & vitamin C).	Confusion, disorientation, easily aroused anger, nervousness, rapid pulse, tremors.
Manganese	Bananas, bran, celery, cereals, egg yolks, green leafy vegetables, legumes, liver, nuts, pineapples, whole grains.	Enzyme activation, reproduction & growth, sex hormone production, tissue respiration, vitamin B1 metabolism, vitamin E utilization.	Ataxia (muscle coordination failure), dizziness, ear noises, loss of hearing.
Phosphorus	Eggs, fish, grains, glandular meats, meat, poultry, yellow cheese, milk/yogurt, eggs (cooked).	Bone/tooth formation, cell growth & repair, energy production, heart muscles contraction, kidney function, metabolism (calcium, sugar), nerve & muscle activity, vitamin utilization.	Appetite loss, fatigue, irregular breathing, nervous disorders, overweight, weight loss.
Potassium	Dates, figs, peaches, tomato juice, blackstrap molasses, peanuts, raisins, seafood, apricots, (dried) bananas, potatoes (baked), sunflower seeds.	Heartbeat, rapid growth, muscle contraction, nerve tranquilization.	Acne, continuous thirst, dry skin, constipation, general weakness, insomnia, muscle damage, nervousness, slow irregular heartbeat, weak reflexes.
Sodium	Salt, milk, cheese, seafood.	Normal cellular fluid level, proper muscle contraction.	Appetite loss, intestinal gas, muscle shrinkage, vomiting, weight loss.
Sulphur	Bran, cheese, clams, eggs, nuts, fish, wheat germ.	Collagen synthesis, body tissue formation.	Not known.
Zinc	Brewer's yeast, liver, seafood, soy beans, spinach, sunflower seeds, mushrooms.	Burn & wound healing, carbohydrate digestion, prostate gland function, reproductive organ growth & development, sex organ growth & maturity, vitamin B1, phosphorus & protein metabolism.	Delayed sexual maturity, fatigue, loss of taste, poor appetite, prolonged wound healing, retarded growth, sterility.

United States Recommended Daily Allowances* For Vitamins And Minerals

Vitamin	Infants	Children 1 to 4 years	Children over 4 and Adults	Pregnant or lactating women
AIU	1500	2500	5000	8000
DIU	400	400	400	400
EIU	5	10	30	30
C mg.	35	40	60	60
Folic acid mcg.	100	200	400	800
Thiamin (B1) mg.	0.5	0.7	1.5	1.7
Riboflavin (B2) mg.	0.6	0.8	1.7	2
Niacin mg.	8	9	20	20
Pyridoxine (B6) mg.	0.4	0.7	2	2.5
Cobalamin (B12) mcg.	2	3	6	8
Biotin mcg.	50	150	300	300
Pantothenic acid mg.	3	5	10	10

Mineral	Infants	Children 1 to 4 years	Children over 4 and Adults	Pregnant or lactating women
Calcium (g)	0.6	0.8	1.0	1.3
Phosphorus (g)	0.5	0.8	1.0	1.3
Iodine (mcg.)	45.0	70.0	150.0	150.0
Iron (mg)	15.0	10.0	18.0	18.0
Magnesium (mg)	70.0	200.0	400.0	450.0
Copper (mg)	0.6	1.0	2.0	2.0
Zinc (mg)	5.0	8.0	15.0	15.0

I.U. = International Units mg. = milligrams mcg. = micrograms

Note: No allowances have yet been determined for vitamin K.

PLEASE NOTE: If, after medical tests, your doctor found that you need vitamin and/or mineral supplements, let him recommend those which you may need.

*USRDA's are set by Federal Food and Drug Administration based on recommended dietary allowances established by the National Research Council—National Academy of Sciences.

Nutritional
Analysis
of Recipes

NUTRITIONAL ANALYSIS TABLES

All recipes are grouped as shown in the Table of Contents and are in alphabetical order within each category. Recipe page numbers are given for your convenience, and individual listings are included in the index. Emergency Rations are identified by "(E)" following applicable entries.

Nutritional information has been limited to those nutrients tested by the United States Department of Agriculture and therefore does not include biotin, copper, folic acid, manganese, pantothenic acid, selenium, vitamins B_6, B_{12}, & E, zinc, etc.

The totals shown reflect averages of the nutrients in the ingredients as tested, *not* the amounts assimilated. It has been suggested that 25 percent to 30 percent be deducted for normal loss in absorption, but in some cases the losses can be much higher. (For vegetable vitamin A, carotene, the loss can range from 99 percent in raw carrots to 65 percent for pureed, cooked carrots.) In all cases, food values and assimilation are subject to many variables, so these tables are intended merely as guides toward a more complete and balanced diet.

Statistics have been compiled from *Composition of Foods, USDA Handbook #8; Dairy & Egg Products, USDA Handbook #8-1; Spices & Herbs, USDA Handbook #8-2; Nutritive Value of Foods, USDA Bulletin #7;* and both the 1975 and 1979 editions of *Nutrition Almanac,* McGraw Hill Paperbacks (GNC #18651).

	Page No.	Nutritional Analysis based on servings as indicated	Food Energy Calories	Protein Grams	Fat Grams	Carbohydrate Grams	Fiber Grams	Calcium Mg	Iron Mg	Magnesium Mg	Phosphorus Mg	Potassium Mg	Sodium Mg	Vitamin A IU	Thiamin B_1 Mg	Riboflavin Mg	Niacin Mg	Vitamin C Mg
SOUPS																		
Cock-a-Leekie	9	1	154	11.8	2.8	21.0	1.1	53	2.5	43	198	505	689	2,096	.18	.11	3.2	142
Cream of Lettuce & Tomato Soup	10	1	124	9.2	3.8	14.0	.6	240	2.0	30	191	532	574	1,565	.12	.29	.6	24
Hotch-Potch	12	1	107	4.1	3.5	15.7	.9	46	1.2	20	78	333	655	3,100	.13	.09	trace	269
Lentil-Barley Soup	14	1	151	7.8	2.3	16.8	1.6	53	2.7	35	126	496	479	1,977	.14	.10	1.3	12
" super-nutrition	15	1	178	11.4	2.7	19.2	1.7	312	3.2	102	213	652	855	2,064	.15	.12	2.1	139
Quick Chili with Beans	16	1	248	20.9	9.0	28.4	1.9	80	5.0	82	301	874	600	802	.16	.23	4.4	17
Root-Cellar Soup	18	1	181	16.0	4.1	20.7	1.4	116	3.4	45	201	524	648	890	.19	.16	3.2	18
Salmon Soup	20	1	240	20.3	8.4	20.5	.5	435	1.2	64	433	631	703	367	.15	.50	5.1	13
" super-nutrition	22	1	242	20.3	8.4	21.0	.5	435	1.3	64	435	631	703	559	1.93	4.00	6.3	146
Vitamin "P" Soup	22	1	186	13.3	4.4	26.2	1.0	164	2.2	75	212	701	590	2,226	.28	.29	1.8	21
" super-nutrition	23	1	209	14.0	6.4	27.0	1.0	172	2.5	82	262	753	603	2,226	.54	.37	2.4	104
SALAD DRESSINGS																		
Almost Mayonnaise	27	1 Tbs	31	1.0	.9	1.9	0	28	.8	3	28	39	97	31	.36	.75	.1	47
Bleu Cheese-Sour Cream Salad Dressing	29	1 Tbs	25	1.0	2.1	.8	0	32	trace	2	24	31	41	68	trace	.03	trace	trace

29	Cottage Cheese Salad Dressing	1 Tbs	23	1.3	1.8	.4	0	11	trace	1	27	11	66	28	.02	.02	trace	46
30	" " Sandwich Spread	1 Tbs	20	1.0	1.4	1.0	trace	9	trace	8	2	5	17	333	.47	.94	.2	34
33	Horseradish Dressing for Cole Slaw	1	7	.7	.3	1.4	trace	32	.1	8	20	69	222	25	.01	trace	trace	125
30	Tropical Salad Dressing	¼ cup	46	.1	0	11.3	trace	11	.4	8	6	38	178	trace	trace	.01	trace	0

SALADS & VEGETABLE ICES

31	Bean Salad with Lentils	1	175	8.3	3.2	30.0	1.9	63	2.7	43	141	405	174	1,981	.12	.08	.8	172
39	Bleu Pear Salad	1	136	4.1	7.6	15.9	1.5	80	.6	29	89	250	129	111	.06	.10	.3	130
32	Chicken Salad Supreme	1	93	9.6	3.1	5.0	.2	34	.9	9	71	184	128	141	.22	.44	2.9	25
32	" " super-nutrition	1	93	9.6	3.1	5.2	.2	40	.9	13	72	215	146	141	1.96	3.94	3.0	25
32	Cole Slaw Mousse	1	68	4.8	1.2	8.8	.5	91	1.0	9	85	232	451	1,782	.24	.48	.3	300
33	Cole Slaw with Horseradish Dressing	1	16	1.2	.3	3.4	.3	50	.2	13	31	156	230	98	.19	.23	.5	143
34	" " super-nutrition	1	16	1.2	.3	3.4	.3	50	.2	13	31	156	230	1,348	1.94	3.73	1.6	168
34	Curried Lobster Salad	1	342	20.2	12.6	34.8	.7	115	3.1	101	337	562	631	534	2.50	4.79	5.6	307
35	Eggplant Antipasto	1	82	1.6	5.5	7.3	.9	30	.8	15	42	247	297	1,785	.07	.06	.7	140
37	Onion Relish Salad	1	35	1.1	.1	8.3	1.0	27	.5	10	27	195	234	982	.05	.07	.6	27
38	" " super-nutrition	(E) 1	35	1.1	.1	8.3	1.0	27	.5	10	27	195	234	2,232	.05	.07	.6	152

Food	Page No.	Nutritional Analysis based on servings as indicated	Food Energy Calories	Protein Grams	Fat Grams	Carbo-hydrate Grams	Fiber Grams	Calcium Mg	Iron Mg	Magnes-ium Mg	Phos-phorus Mg	Potas-sium Mg	Sodium Mg	Vitamin A IU	Thiamin B₁ Mg	Ribo-flavin Mg	Niacin Mg	Vitamin C Mg
Pear-Crabmeat Salad	38	1	175	11.4	8.4	16.1	1.5	98	.9	43	163	296	254	1,033	.12	.13	1.5	131
Potato Salad	39	1 cup	207	9.5	6.5	21.7	.9	117	1.8	46	202	630	562	834	1.09	2.14	1.7	162
" super-nutrition	39	1 cup	213	10.0	6.5	22.4	.9	176	1.8	67	216	654	570	1,668	2.26	4.49	2.5	245
Tropical Garbanzo Salad	40	1	196	6.3	5.8	32.1	2.2	60	2.5	46	112	451	120	2,557	.16	.12	1.2	278
" super-nutrition	41	1	226	7.3	7.8	34.1	2.2	110	2.6	76	200	451	120	2,707	2.04	3.62	2.4	278
Tuna Salad	41	(E) 1	168	17.7	6.6	3.7	.1	58	2.4	42	174	264	582	2,866	2.45	4.97	8.7	197
Vegetable Ices, Celery	43	1	42	1.2	trace	9.9	.1	15	.1	3	10	116	286	135	.01	.03	.2	170
" Cocktail	45	1	52	1.6	.1	12.0	.3	15	.6	1	18	175	408	704	.03	.04	.4	184
" Cucumber-Dill	42	1	43	1.3	trace	10.0	.3	15	.5	6	12	80	252	156	.01	.03	.1	171
" Piquant-Carrot	44	1	77	1.7	.3	17.7	.7	30	.7	21	28	253	371	4,240	.03	.04	.4	171
" Tomato	44	1	51	1.6	.1	11.5	.3	15	.6	13	17	154	273	704	.03	.04	.4	183
" Zucchini-Mint	43	1	44	1.4	trace	10.2	.2	19	.3	8	14	100	250	203	.02	.05	.4	174
CHEESES & DIPS, APPETIZERS & SNACKS																		
Caraway Cheese Spread	55	(E) 2Tbs	73	4.7	5.3	2.2	.3	62	.5	27	48	84	210	1,213	1.28	2.54	.6	83

Cheddar-Olive Spread or Dip	56	(E) 2 Tbs	82	4.3	5.8	2.4	.3	98	.8	12	93	92	195	730	.80	1.61	.6	72
Spicy Egg & Olive Spread or Dip	57	(E) 2 Tbs	81	4.5	6.2	2.2	.3	102	.8	13	91	99	133	3,783	.03	.08	.1	trace
" with optionals	57	(E) 2 Tbs	81	4.5	6.2	2.2	.3	102	.8	13	91	99	133	3,783	.96	1.95	.4	63
Walnut-Soy Spread or Dip	58	(E) 2 Tbs	88	3.7	7.5	2.1	.2	80	.6	12	81	83	201	202	.03	.03	.1	trace
" with optionals	58	(E) 2 Tbs	88	3.7	7.5	2.1	.2	80	.6	12	81	83	201	827	.91	1.78	.7	75
Cucumber Dip	53	2 Tbs	19	2.3	.7	1.0	.1	52	.2	24	21	44	111	932	.01	.03	.4	86
Garbanzo-Sesame Dip	58	2 Tbs	80	3.4	4.5	7.6	.7	25	.9	24	78	125	196	15	.05	.02	.6	trace
" super-nutrition	60	2 Tbs	80	3.4	4.5	7.6	.7	25	.9	24	78	125	196	1,015	.75	1.42	1.1	118
Chicken Liver Pâté	60	2 Tbs	61	4.0	4.4	1.6	trace	14	1.4	7	46	97	120	1,736	.04	.34	1.4	.3
" super-nutrition	61	2 Tbs	62	4.0	4.5	1.8	trace	17	1.4	9	63	112	111	1,678	.97	2.22	2.7	127
Snack Crackers—Cheddar	64	(E) 10	75	3.4	5.0	4.6	.1	79	.3	12	79	28	125	144	.04	.05	.3	0
" with optional B-complex	64	(E) 10	75	3.4	5.0	4.6	.1	79	.3	12	79	28	125	144	.46	.88	.4	0
Snack Crackers—Celery Seed	62	(E) 10	69	1.5	3.9	7.4	.2	14	.4	15	47	32	122	111	.06	.02	.3	0
" super-nutrition	64	(E) 10	78	3.9	3.9	7.5	.2	46	.4	29	66	43	129	565	.75	1.43	1.0	0

ENTRIES—MEATS	Page No.	Nutritional Analysis based on servings as indicated	Food Energy Calories	Protein Grams	Fat Grams	Carbohydrate Grams	Fiber Grams	Calcium Mg	Iron Mg	Magnesium Mg	Phosphorus Mg	Potassium Mg	Sodium Mg	Vitamin A IU	Thiamin B_1 Mg	Riboflavin Mg	Niacin Mg	Vitamin C Mg
Beef Breakfast Sausage	71	1	123	12.3	7.5	1.4	.3	18	2.0	13	131	244	383	40	.08	.11	2.8	250
" super-nutrition	72	1	168	14.1	10.9	3.9	.4	148	2.3	81	244	311	421	1,585	.23	.13	2.8	250
Beef Sausage w/Limas, w/o supplements	73	1 of 6	271	17.1	10.4	28.6	1.7	53	4.5	66	255	789	665	126	.27	.15	2.4	2
" complete meal for 6	73	1	438	24.0	16.1	56.3	3.9	182	6.2	118	399	1,354	1,130	3,365	.47	.42	4.4	274
Breaded Calves' Liver	80	1	289	25.0	13.3	16.6	.1	57	10.5	19	436	437	231	25,841	.64	3.84	13.8	93
Depression Goulash	76	1	365	26.0	17.8	22.5	1.0	254	4.0	63	333	571	517	1,923	.30	.40	5.5	23
" super-nutrition	78	1	384	26.7	19.2	24.0	1.0	292	4.0	86	392	591	529	2,023	1.63	2.91	6.0	189
Double Bean & Beef w/o rice or lettuce	75	1	215	20.5	10.2	14.9	1.6	108	4.5	62	255	668	1,160	595	.22	.29	3.8	9
" super-nutrition	76	1	215	20.5	10.2	14.9	1.6	108	4.5	62	255	668	1,160	1,845	1.97	3.79	4.9	159
Good Old Meat Loaf	69	1	233	22.9	9.9	10.9	.8	152	4.0	57	340	623	385	715	.33	.36	4.7	1
" super-nutrition	70	1	245	23.3	10.7	11.7	.8	221	4.0	92	375	623	385	2,775	3.38	6.36	5.7	108
Great Northern Casserole	85	4	252	27.6	3.8	27.0	1.7	90	4.9	61	365	981	435	804	.21	.28	8.0	64
" super-nutrition	86	1	252	27.6	3.8	27.0	1.7	151	4.9	90	365	981	435	2,055	2.08	4.03	8.6	154
" variation w/ lima beans	86	1	266	27.9	3.8	30.1	1.7	136	5.2	101	369	1,121	432	2,055	2.08	4.02	8.6	154

Item	Page																	
"Instant" Swiss Steak	78	1	273	33.2	11.3	10.2	.4	57	6.6	67	364	811	517	497	.46	.36	8.2	trace
" super-nutrition	79	1	273	33.2	11.3	10.2	.4	57	6.6	67	364	811	517	497	2.21	3.86	9.3	307
Lamb with Artichoke Hearts	80	1	240	22.8	12.4	7.0	1.5	50	2.7	inc.	239	544	503	94	.23	.29	6.7	trace
" super-nutrition	81	1	240	22.8	12.4	7.2	1.5	56	2.7	inc.	240	574	520	1,344	.23	.31	6.7	125
Oriental Pork, Indoor BBQ	82	1	432	20.5	11.6	12.7	0	26	3.7	13	237	482	864	1,784	.98	.27	5.4	197
Pork Chop Pilaf	83	1	286	23.2	10.7	24.7	.9	44	3.8	47	308	437	445	284	.82	.35	5.6	37
" super-nutrition	84	1	304	24.5	11.3	26.8	1.9	177	4.1	117	330	555	450	1,663	2.72	4.12	6.4	38
Pot au Feu plus Broth	86	1	356	45.1	10.6	39.0	2.0	97	7.1	108	529	1,175	914	6,285	.35	.65	13.5	trace
Sunflower-Mushroom Meatloaf	70	1	266	22.6	14.7	14.0	.7	148	3.8	62	366	683	417	140	.21	.53	4.5	trace
" super-nutrition	71	1	275	23.9	14.7	15.4	.7	322	4.4	150	425	766	352	140	5.75	10.69	7.5	trace
ENTREES—POULTRY																		
Alfalfa Sprout Egg Fu Yong	90	1	226	17.4	13.1	10.2	.8	104	2.6	47	261	284	715	943	2.11	4.02	4.0	150
" meal with brown rice & tomatoes	91	1	332	20.1	13.8	32.8	1.0	123	3.4	80	336	519	928	1,618	2.23	4.05	5.5	167
Chicken & Broccoli Royale	93	1	315	18.9	18.1	15.9	.9	120	1.7	36	264	400	542	1,812	.08	.21	5.0	53
" super-nutrition	93	1	315	18.9	18.1	15.9	.9	365	1.7	153	264	400	542	4,312	3.80	7.71	6.3	178
Chicken & Noodles, Italian Style	93	1	242	85	6.5	26.3	.5	187	2.0	45	325	551	303	363	.20	.47	5.4	10
" super-nutrition	95	1	252	18.8	7.2	26.9	.5	203	2.0	55	354	551	303	2,080	1.41	2.81	6.2	95

	Page No.	Nutritional Analysis based on servings as indicated	Food Energy Calories	Protein Grams	Fat Grams	Carbo-hydrate Grams	Fiber Grams	Calcium Mg	Iron Mg	Magnes-ium Mg	Phos-phorus Mg	Potas-sium Mg	Sodium Mg	Vitamin A IU	Thiamin B1 Mg	Ribo-flavin Mg	Niacin Mg	Vitamin C Mg
City Chicken Dinner	95	1	263	36.5	2.8	23.1	1.7	64	3.4	82	434	743	392	874	.25	.38	13.6	13
" super-nutrition	96	1	263	36.5	2.8	23.1	1.7	126	3.4	110	434	743	392	2,124	2.00	3.88	14.8	163
Delicatessen Chicken without broth	100	1	226	29.5	4.9	.7	.2	22	1.7	22	149	317	171	1,999	1.92	3.93	10.1	125
Main Dish Millet Pilaf	99	1	209	14.3	6.5	26.3	1.3	31	3.3	60	210	391	631	197	.26	.31	4.6	trace
Mediterranean Chicken Dinner	97	1	278	21.0	6.1	35.5	2.5	117	4.2	49	312	660	534	1,711	.25	.19	5.4	183
ENTREES—SEAFOOD																		
Avocado Tuna Amandine	103	1	439	24.4	21.3	41.0	1.3	244	2.5	125	362	818	1,001	307	.22	.44	8.3	10
Creole Jambalaya	106	1	325	24.5	8.7	38.2	1.3	89	4.2	94	303	808	609	1,480	.36	.20	6.6	52
" super-nutrition	108	1	325	24.6	8.7	40.7	1.3	93	4.2	97	304	832	621	1,586	1.53	2.37	7.4	236
Fillet of Sole, Della Robbia, w/o dressing	104	1	155	22.9	1.2	15.5	.8	42	1.9	50	249	651	217	2,106	.11	.11	2.5	150
" with Bleu Cheese Dressing		1	206	25.0	5.2	16.9	.8	106	2.0	54	297	713	299	2,214	.12	.17	2.6	150
Nut Crusted Trout	108	1	466	32.2	32.7	11.5	.6	72	3.0	inc	inc	745	172	494	.49	.66	10.4	0
Salmon Newburg with Peas	109	1	292	18.8	18.3	14.2	.7	31	2.1	74	431	433	566	1,153	.32	.30	5.2	140
" w/waffle, broccoli & tomato		1	569	34.8	28.0	48.5	2.9	291	5.5	143	879	1,202	968	4,266	1.03	1.19	8.5	240

Tuna Sandwiches	41	1	426	27.0	11.3	33.9	1.2	212	5.8	137	444	566	975	3,998	5.91	9.09	12.8	229
Tuna-Stuffed Tomatoes	41	1	203	19.5	6.9	11.2	.9	84	3.3	68	224	656	584	4,256	2.54	5.00	10.6	232
ENTREES—VEGETARIAN																		
Avocado Amandine	104	1	516	20.1	30.7	45.0	1.5	423	2.4	115	382	788	783	1,334	.26	.61	2.9	10
Blackeyed Jambalaya	107	1	237	9.5	6.2	38.2	1.2	66	3.3	76	217	724	521	1,215	.44	.22	3.7	55
Imperial Pottage	113	1	300	16.0	6.4	52.3	3.1	102	4.7	87	247	706	274	546	.33	.18	2.1	33
" " super-nutrition	115	1	300	16.1	6.4	52.5	3.1	109	4.7	91	248	737	291	1,797	2.08	3.68	3.2	183
Macaroni & Cheese	111	1	377	18.7	22.1	27.6	.3	376	2.3	51	379	242	707	2,154	.22	.52	2.5	8
" " super-nutrition	112	1	387	19.5	22.7	28.6	.4	394	2.6	55	408	257	731	2,202	1.19	2.40	3.3	70
Mediterranean Dinner	99	1	279	13.6	10.1	37.2	2.7	119	3.8	60	260	619	527	1,679	.24	.18	2.0	183
Onion Quiche	115	1	343	11.2	24.4	24.1	.8	227	1.5	45	231	293	509	629	.84	1.53	1.4	7
" " super-nutrition	116	1	360	15.5	24.4	24.1	.8	240	1.5	48	265	293	509	2,296	2.09	4.10	2.5	174
Pepita-Cheese Crepes with sauce	173	2 crepes	458	28.1	27.5	27.3	.6	441	3.2	85	540	424	1,069	1,868	.43	.51	2.0	trace
" " super-nutrition	173	2 crepes	488	29.1	29.5	29.7	.6	503	3.3	123	630	484	1,103	2,018	2.31	4.04	3.2	155
Sunflower-Millet Patties	117	1	256	14.8	13.1	22.6	1.9	215	3.3	52	435	489	420	256	.65	.35	1.8	9
" " super-nutrition	118	1	293	16.8	15.1	25.6	1.9	270	3.8	88	566	536	424	2,906	1.18	.45	2.7	134

	Page No.	Nutritional Analysis based on servings as indicated	Food Energy Calories	Protein Grams	Fat Grams	Carbo-hydrate Grams	Fiber Grams	Calcium Mg	Iron Mg	Magnes-ium Mg	Phos-phorus Mg	Potas-sium Mg	Sodium Mg	Vitamin A IU	Thiamin B_1 Mg	Ribo-flavin Mg	Niacin Mg	Vitamin C Mg
Swiss Potatoes & Onions	118	1	305	15.0	15.4	27.6	.9	458	1.2	72	389	580	657	535	.37	.35	1.6	24
" " super-nutrition	120	1	305	15.0	15.4	27.6	.9	458	1.2	72	389	580	657	1,785	2.12	3.85	2.7	174
Vegetarian Egg Fu Yong	91	1	205	10.6	13.9	11.5	1.1	164	2.8	74	300	261	631	877	2.12	4.06	1.9	150
VEGETABLES																		
Corn Cakes	142	1	158	6.8	6.9	18.3	.5	89	1.3	43	147	265	307	682	.46	.71	1.3	62
Cucumber-Onion Stir-Fry	143	1	64	1.0	3.6	7.8	.5	24	.8	11	26	138	392	1,371	.02	.03	.1	258
Golden Delicious Limas	130	1	238	8.4	4.2	44.0	2.5	44	3.4	87	167	701	282	198	.16	.08	.8	255
" " with optionals	131	1	238	8.4	4.2	44.0	2.5	44	3.4	87	167	701	282	1,448	2.03	3.84	1.5	255
Herbed Carrots	140	1	66	1.2	3.0	8.7	.9	41	.8	21	33	2,915	208	9,500	.05	.04	.5	132
Kidney Beans with Pears (Baked)	128	1	132	5.2	.7	27.5	1.4	38	1.9	38	102	300	129	122	.04	.05	.6	2
" " super-nutrition	129	1	129	5.2	.7	27.0	1.4	69	2.6	49	105	438	133	1,372	1.80	3.56	1.8	277
Minted Celery	142	1	46	1.2	2.9	4.6	.6	49	.6	21	32	300	329	366	.02	.03	.1	133
Parsnip Patties	144	1	122	5.1	4.0	17.5	1.7	83	1.1	38	126	583	182	186	.10	.19	.3	6
Scalloped Potatoes	144	1	170	6.6	3.2	27.3	.8	129	1.2	50	163	659	298	353	.35	.56	2.2	51

Food	Page	Serving																
Soybean Meat Extender (pulp from Soymilk)	136	½ cup	71	5.3	3.0	7.6	1.4	37	1.3	10	95	239	0	0	.21	.05	.4	0
Soymilk—home enriched	137	1 cup	113	11.6	3.5	8.9	0	309	1.9	159	245	511	57	1,345	.22	.26	.6	0
Soy Succotash	135	1	148	7.9	8.5	12.2	1.0	93	1.6	43	145	340	452	164	.20	1.00	.8	4
Spring Skillet	141	1	64	1.3	3.0	8.9	1.2	45	.9	18	38	295	320	7,278	.05	.06	.6	145
Stuffed Baked Potatoes	145	1	185	7.1	4.0	30.9	.9	40	1.1	48	132	104	218	258	.15	.12	2.4	256
Sweet & Sour Beans	129	1	247	9.7	1.9	50.3	2.4	60	3.4	74	178	561	290	1,602	.19	.12	1.1	296
20th Century Baked Beans	127	1	164	8.7	1.0	31.4	1.6	101	4.1	56	175	678	186	190	.17	.10	1.1	148
" super-nutrition #1	128	1	164	8.7	1.0	31.4	1.6	101	4.1	56	175	678	186	1,440	2.04	3.85	1.7	148
" super-nutrition #2, w/soybeans	128	1	177	12.1	6.4	20.5	1.8	126	4.1	117	207	810	180	222	.24	.12	1.4	148
Yam & Peanut Boats	146	1	310	9.8	15.4	33.8	1.6	68	1.2	96	205	961	190	11,719	.19	.13	4.9	31

CONDIMENTS, SAUCES & SYRUPS

Food	Page	Serving																
Almost Sour Cream & Chives	161	2 Tbs	22	3.4	.5	1.0	trace	34	.1	2	47	35	102	79	.01	.05	trace	101
Rotisserie Magic	155	1	23	.2	2.4	.7	.2	11	.3	6	4	51	171	1,744	1.88	3.78	.7	125
Seasoned Flour	154	2 Tbs	60	2.7	.4	11.2	.1	28	.6	13	43	94	145	301	.41	.74	.8	53
Instant Ketchup, with optionals	156	1 Tbs	11	.2	.5	1.6	trace	8	.3	4	10	77	54	176	.01	.03	.2	46

Food	Page No.	Nutritional Analysis based on servings as indicated	Food Energy Calories	Protein Grams	Fat Grams	Carbo-hydrate Grams	Fiber Grams	Calcium Mg	Iron Mg	Magnes-ium Mg	Phos-phorus Mg	Potas-sium Mg	Sodium Mg	Vitamin A IU	Thiamin B₁ Mg	Ribo-flavin Mg	Niacin Mg	Vitamin C Mg
Mushroom Ketchup	157	1 Tbs	9	.3	.3	1.4	.1	8	.3	5	15	88	85	78	.05	.07	.5	62
Quick & Easy Tomato Sauce	158	¼ cup	45	1.5	1.9	6.3	.3	16	1.3	13	44	302	149	900	.06	.06	.9	116
Fresh Tomato Sauce	159	¼ cup	37	1.6	1.3	5.7	.3	19	1.2	17	52	295	199	828	.18	.09	1.1	83
Mexican Chili-Cheese Sauce	160	¼ cup	46	3.7	4.0	4.8	.3	84	1.0	16	90	214	233	776	.21	.13	1.6	58
Mushroom Tomato Sauce	159	¼ cup	35	1.7	1.3	5.1	.3	19	1.3	13	63	305	183	450	.19	.14	2.2	78
Slow & Easy Tomato Sauce	160	¼ cup	25	1.1	.6	4.3	.4	21	.9	12	18	215	247	1,019	.04	.03	.6	13
" " with meat & mushrooms		¼ cup	32	2.5	.9	3.9	.4	19	1.0	12	37	220	235	892	.04	.05	.9	11
Swiss Cream Sauce	171	1	135	6.0	9.1	9.7	trace	153	.6	17	133	153	385	179	.06	.15	.4	0
Curried Peaches & Pears	162	1	64	.4	2.0	9.9	.6	7	.3	6	10	101	104	462	.01	.03	.5	3
" " super-nutrition	163	1	84	.6	2.0	10.4	.7	12	.6	8	17	153	106	1,298	1.27	2.53	1.0	86
Fig Dessert Sauce	164	1	153	2.5	.6	35.3	.9	82	.6	16	60	197	30	29	.11	.11	.5	167
Ginger Peachy Sauce	164	1	159	1.0	5.9	26.9	.4	17	.6	20	29	192	65	590	.08	.04	.6	184
Nutty Nectarine Sauce	163	1	166	1.3	5.4	29.3	.3	17	.6	22	36	212	67	691	.06	.03	.4	186
Almost Maple Syrup	165	1 Tbs	28	0	0	7.7	0	5	.2	3	1	21	1	trace	trace	trace	trace	0

BREADS — CREPES

Basic Crepes	169	1 crepe	64	3.4	2.9	6.1	.2	39	.6	13	65	61	66	192	.05	.09	.5	trace
Spinach-Chicken Pepita Crepes w/sauce	170	2 crepes	464	28.5	29.0	26.3	.8	371	3.6	62	496	551	812	1,882	.32	.55	5.5	5
" super-nutrition	173	2 crepes	495	28.8	31.0	26.6	.8	434	3.8	102	600	627	847	2,032	2.33	4.10	7.0	155

BREADS — PANCAKES & WAFFLES

Old Fashioned Buckwheat Pancakes	174	1 cake	87	3.7	1.9	15.2	.6	56	.6	33	83	117	110	54	.06	.09	.7	trace
" super-nutrition	175	1 cake	101	4.7	3.0	16.0	.8	126	1.0	78	166	158	111	129	.30	.14	1.3	trace
Yeast Waffles — Basic	175	1 waffle	200	8.4	7.5	24.9	.4	138	1.5	60	260	226	162	250	.50	.30	2.0	0
" Corn	179	1 waffle	253	10.5	11.3	29.2	.6	180	1.2	82	322	266	353	462	.33	.23	1.4	2
" Oatmeal	177	1 waffle	240	12.4	9.3	27.5	.5	166	2.3	38	372	380	391	163	.59	.55	2.2	0
" Sugar-Honey Graham	180	1 waffle	313	11.1	14.5	36.2	.6	157	2.0	60	301	386	360	525	.54	.38	2.2	trace

BREADS — MUFFINS & CORNBREAD

Regulation Muffins	185	1 muffin	121	4.3	4.5	17.8	.8	93	1.5	39	147	272	117	188	.14	.13	1.0	trace
Carrot Cornbread	186	1	145	5.0	5.7	19.4	.4	87	.8	30	118	180	253	1,594	.10	.13	.4	1
" super-nutrition	187	1	156	5.8	6.2	20.4	.4	132	1.0	55	161	203	255	1,631	.33	.18	.9	1
Wheat-Free Yeast Cornbread	187	1	136	5.1	4.5	19.2	.2	87	.8	45	165	145	150	220	.18	.13	.4	trace

	Page No.	Nutritional Analysis based on servings as indicated	Food Energy Calories	Protein Grams	Fat Grams	Carbohydrate Grams	Fiber Grams	Calcium Mg	Iron Mg	Magnesium Mg	Phosphorus Mg	Potassium Mg	Sodium Mg	Vitamin A IU	Thiamin B₁ Mg	Riboflavin Mg	Niacin Mg	Vitamin C Mg
BREADS — POCKET BREADS																		
All-Star Protein Pocket Bread	183	1	143	10.9	2.7	24.6	.5	26	1.2	33	168	110	244	0	inc	inc	inc	0
Basic Wheat Pocket Bread	181	1	168	5.5	2.7	31.3	.6	15	1.5	37	157	134	244	0	.29	.17	2.4	0
" super-nutrition	182	1	168	5.5	2.7	31.3	.6	56	1.5	56	157	134	244	0	1.46	2.40	3.1	17
Cornmeal Pocket Breads	183	1	175	5.9	2.8	31.8	.5	12	1.2	32	129	111	244	47	inc	inc	inc	0
Gluten Pocket Breads	183	1	168	7.3	2.8	29.3	.6	14	1.3	36	155	130	244	0	inc	inc	inc	0
Rye Pocket Breads	184	1	166	6.2	2.9	30.4	.7	26	2.0	40	195	274	244	trace	.30	.19	1.0	0
BREADS — LOAF BREADS & ROLLS																		
All-Star Protein Bread	201	1 slice	70	6.3	1.2	8.6	.2	73	.6	29	106	105	124	trace	.19	.14	1.0	trace
Beginning Rye Bread	193	1 slice	82	3.2	1.0	15.8	.4	18	1.1	21	95	156	99	trace	.22	.10	1.1	0
Beginning Wheat Bread	189	1 slice	98	3.4	1.2	18.6	.3	23	.8	17	65	80	115	trace	.15	.11	1.5	0
Golden Glow Bread	195	1 slice	97	3.5	2.0	17.1	.4	12	1.3	19	70	111	113	1,163	.11	.06	1.1	trace
" super-nutrition	196	1 slice	98	3.7	1.9	17.3	.4	41	1.4	33	86	123	114	1,181	1.04	1.75	2.4	trace
Rice-Bran Wheat Bread	196	1 slice	119	4.3	2.2	21.6	.5	28	1.1	27	103	79	163	trace	.16	.13	1.4	2
" super-nutrition	198	1 slice	118	4.4	2.1	21.5	.5	65	1.4	44	119	119	164	556	1.05	1.81	2.7	2

Sandwich Buns	206	1 med	190	7.1	4.2	31.2	.4	61	1.5	34	124	199	271	3	.41	.27	2.5	0
" super-nutrition	207	1 med	182	7.2	4.2	29.8	.6	83	1.5	51	146	218	271	3	1.02	1.49	2.5	0
Sesame Egg Bread	198	1 slice	91	4.3	1.8	15.4	.4	67	.9	22	95	113	127	37	.13	.11	.9	trace
" super-nutrition	200	1 slice	98	4.5	2.5	15.6	.4	95	1.0	36	111	124	128	37	.63	.96	1.3	trace
Tender-Crust Rolls	203	1	155	4.4	7.1	22.5	.3	38	1.0	24	111	121	207	253	.28	.16	1.6	trace
Steamed Brown Bread	208	1 slice	55	2.5	.5	11.0	.2	60	1.1	26	77	230	68	9	.14	.10	.7	trace
Steamed Date-Nut Bread	211	1 slice	77	2.5	2.0	13.4	.3	61	1.1	34	92	204	47	50	.15	.08	.6	trace

DESSERTS — ICE CREAM & FROZEN DESSERTS

Almost Ice Cream	216	1	124	6.2	5.6	12.4	0	169	.3	29	143	127	138	258	.05	.23	.1	50
Old-Fashioned Custard Ice Cream	215	1	165	4.7	11.3	11.7	0	145	.3	33	108	140	89	480	.04	.15	trace	50
Mission Sherbet	165	1	243	3.9	.9	56.0	1.4	126	1.0	30	97	357	45	105	.19	.18	.7	266
Frozen Dessert Crepes	222	1 crepe	144	5.1	3.1	25.0	.6	82	1.1	30	110	312	83	953	.08	.15	.7	176

DESSERTS — PUDDINGS, PIE FILLINGS & FRUIT DESSERTS

Caramel Pudding	217	1	306	6.6	10.9	52.7	trace	217	2.7	62	180	549	413	2,897	.07	.26	.5	trace
" with Banana	219	1	348	7.2	11.0	63.8	.3	221	3.0	79	-193	734	413	2,992	.10	.29	.8	6
" with Carob	218	1	328	7.2	11.1	62.8	1.0	261	2.7	62	200	549	413	2,897	.07	.26	.5	trace

	Page No.	Nutritional Analysis based on servings as indicated	Food Energy Calories	Protein Grams	Fat Grams	Carbohydrate Grams	Fiber Grams	Calcium Mg	Iron Mg	Magnesium Mg	Phosphorus Mg	Potassium Mg	Sodium Mg	Vitamin A IU	Thiamin B_1 Mg	Riboflavin Mg	Niacin Mg	Vitamin C Mg
Chunky Pineapple-Pear Pudding or Pie Filling	224	1	111	5.2	1.3	21.1	.9	106	.5	18	88	202	59	142	.08	.19	.2	173
" super-nutrition w/fructose	225	1	128	9.5	1.3	21.1	.9	161	.5	40	121	202	59	1,809	.08	.26	.9	173
Nectarine-Grape Mousse	219	1	87	2.3	.4	19.3	.3	32	.4	9	38	244	38	894	.11	.05	.3	16
" super-nutrition	220	1	92	2.9	.5	19.9	.3	35	.7	12	67	275	40	2,560	.37	.12	1.0	183
Sultan's Delight—Fig Pudding	220	1	273	9.2	10.2	45.4	3.1	153	1.2	54	156	368	199	49	.22	.14	3.8	trace
Honey Baked Pears	221	1	143	2.2	4.5	25.5	1.4	20	.9	26	60	230	5	21	.09	.06	.3	128
Snow-Capped Pears	222	1	213	4.7	5.8	44.0	2.7	78	1.2	33	79	275	30	21	.09	.10	.3	128
DESSERTS — PIES																		
Apple Meringue Pie	232	1	420	9.7	15.9	65.3	.9	145	2.7	46	226	444	304	1,262	.87	1.57	1.7	169
Bartlett Pie Tart	228	1 of 6	304	4.0	14.8	40.7	1.1	31	1.6	32	93	193	360	646	.19	.12	1.2	2
" super-nutrition	230	1 of 6	324	4.7	16.2	42.0	1.1	146	1.6	91	151	193	360	746	1.53	2.62	1.6	169
Green Tomato Pie	231	1	483	7.3	25.4	61.6	1.2	96	2.5	92	237	397	377	535	1.68	2.64	3.0	184
Lime Cream Pie	226	1	475	16.7	22.1	57.0	.9	165	1.5	56	288	262	438	76	1.96	2.84	3.1	178

Item	Page	Serving																
Maple Nut Pie, without garnish	227	1	473	9.3	34.4	53.9	1.4	244	2.5	70	250	670	277	10,895	.94	1.56	1.9	8
" " super-nutrition	228	1	491	9.3	36.4	53.9	1.4	244	2.5	71	271	670	277	10,895	2.10	3.90	2.7	191
Wheat Pastry, single crust	223	1 of 6	145	2.4	10.0	12.9	.3	15	.6	20	65	51	81	25	.75	1.30	1.1	0

DESSERTS — CAKES, FROSTINGS & TOPPINGS

Item	Page	Serving																
Apple-Layer Date Cake	234	(E) 1	185	6.0	7.9	20.6	.8	92	1.6	52	149	339	83	772	.35	.22	1.8	11
" with Date Topping	236	(E) 1	212	6.5	9.5	22.2	.9	108	1.8	55	163	384	113	840	.36	.25	2.0	43
Brown Velvet Cake, unfrosted	238	1	228	6.0	6.9	37.2	.5	80	1.5	23	105	248	276	312	.16	.20	1.2	2
" " super-nutrition	240	1	242	6.0	8.5	37.3	.5	111	1.5	38	121	248	276	937	1.03	1.95	1.8	127
Caramel Spice Cake with Caramel Topping	237	1	382	6.4	17.0	54.1	.7	135	2.2	65	177	343	224	1,458	.21	.14	.9	trace
Honey White Cake, unfrosted	243	1	260	4.2	10.9	37.2	.1	75	.7	11	50	84	199	trace	.14	.16	1.2	trace
Lo-Carb Angel Food Cake, unfrosted	242	1	57	3.7	.1	10.0	trace	4	.3	5	12	45	97	0	.06	.11	.5	125
" " super-nutrition	243	1	57	3.7	.1	10.0	trace	66	.3	19	26	45	97	0	.06	.11	.5	125
Seed Cake-Caraway, plain	242	1	119	3.1	5.1	16.0	.2	50	.8	10	70	65	100	173	.08	.09	.6	trace
" Poppy Seed, plain	240	1	122	2.8	5.7	15.6	.2	68	.6	14	75	69	101	170	.09	.09	.5	trace
" with Brown Sugar Glaze	241	1	139	2.8	5.9	19.4	.2	68	.8	14	75	69	119	179	.10	.10	.5	28
Fruit & Nut Filling	245	1	104	2.0	4.1	16.6	.4	48	.6	15	50	138	32	6	.03	.06	.2	31
" " super-nutrition	246	1	111	2.1	4.6	17.1	.4	61	.6	22	72	138	32	662	.50	.93	.5	37

	Page No.	Nutritional Analysis based on servings as indicated	Food Energy Calories	Protein Grams	Fat Grams	Carbo-hydrate Grams	Fiber Grams	Calcium Mg	Iron Mg	Magnes-ium Mg	Phos-phorus Mg	Potas-sium Mg	Sodium Mg	Vitamin A IU	Thiamin B₁ Mg	Ribo-flavin Mg	Niacin Mg	Vitamin C Mg
Honey Fluff Frosting	246	1	63	.5	0	16.7	0	1	.1	trace	2	16	22	0	trace	.02	.1	31
Maple Fluff Frosting	246	1	52	.5	0	12.8	0	33	.2	trace	4	32	24	0	trace	trace	trace	31
Marshmallow Frosting	246	1	36	.7	0	8.8	0	trace	trace	trace	trace	8	6	0	trace	.01	trace	62
Whipped Topping #1, skim milk powder	247	3 Tbs	19	1.9	0	2.7	0	58	trace	11	96	179	41	4	.04	.01	trace	167
Whipped Topping #2, banana	248	3 Tbs	17	.8	0	3.7	trace	2	.1	trace	5	69	8	32	trace	.02	trace	85
DESSERTS —COOKIES & CANDIES																		
"Chocolate Chip" Cookies	248	(E) 1 cookie	86	1.8	4.2	12.1	.3	37	.4	22	43	51	56	416	.07	.03	.2	trace
Fruit & Nut Bonbons	250	(E) 4 bonbons	238	6.8	13.1	31.5	2.1	71	2.1	54	193	363	50	17	.26	.09	2.0	trace
super-nutrition	250	(E) 4 bonbons	238	6.8	13.1	31.5	2.1	152	2.1	93	193	363	50	851	.89	1.34	2.2	83